# ACSM Fitness Book

## Third Edition

D0958936

*American College of Sports Medicine*

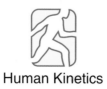

Human Kinetics

**Library of Congress Cataloging-in-Publication Data**

ACSM fitness book / American College of Sports Medicine. -- 3rd ed.
   p.    cm.
   Includes index.
   0-7360-4406-X
   1. Exercise.   2. Physical fitness--Testing.   I. Title: Fitness book.
II. Title: American College of Sports Medicine fitness book.   III.
American College of Sports Medicine.
   GV481 .A322   2002
   613.7'1--dc21

                                        2002008864
ISBN: 0-7360-4406-X

**Acquisitions Editor:** Edward McNeely; **Managing Editor:** Wendy McLaughlin; **Assistant Editor:** Kim Thoren; **Copyeditor:** NOVA Graphic Services; **Proofreader:** Joanna Hatzopoulos Portman; **Indexer:** Marie Rizzo; **Permission Manager:** Toni Harte; **Graphic Designer:** Fred Starbird; **Cover Designer:** Jack W. Davis; **Photographer (cover):** © Corbis; **Photographer (interior):** Carl Johnson; **Art and Photo Managers:** Carl Johnson, Dan Wendt; **Illustrators:** Patrick Griffin, Dick Flood; **ACSM Group Publisher:** D. Mark Robertson

Human Kinetics books are available at special discounts for bulk purchase. Special editions or book excerpts can also be created to specification. For details, contact the Special Sales Manager at Human Kinetics.

Printed in Hong Kong by Creative Printing USA    10  9  8  7  6  5  4  3  2  1

**Human Kinetics**
Web site: http://www.HumanKinetics.com/

*United States:* Human Kinetics
P.O. Box 5076
Champaign, IL 61825-5076
800-747-4457
e-mail: humank@hkusa.com

*Canada:* Human Kinetics
475 Devonshire Road Unit 100
Windsor, ON  N8Y 2L5
800-465-7301 (in Canada only)
e-mail: orders@hkcanada.com

*Europe:* Human Kinetics
107 Bradford Road
Stanningley
Leeds LS28 6AT, United Kingdom
+44 (0) 113 255 5665
e-mail: hk@hkeurope.com

*Australia:* Human Kinetics
57A Price Avenue
Lower Mitcham, South Australia 5062
08 8277 1555
e-mail: liahka@senet.com.au

*New Zealand:* Human Kinetics
P.O. Box 105-231, Auckland Central
09-523-3462
e-mail: hkp@ihug.co.nz

# Contents

# Foreword

Since the publication of my own first book, *Pumping Iron* (1974), and my second book with Douglas Kent Hall, *The Education of a Body Builder* (1977), I have been an open advocate for physical fitness. President George H.W. Bush had sufficient confidence in my proactive stance toward fitness that he named me the Chairman of the President's Council on Physical Fitness in 1990. During the time I served on the President's Council, I traveled to all 50 States advocating physical fitness. My advocacy continued when I was named the Chairman of the California Governor's Council on Physical Fitness. As I travel around the country today, I am still concerned about the poor state of physical fitness for such a large segment of the population, especially the fitness level of our kids. I continue to be an advocate for fitness in my position as the Chairman of the Board of the Inner-City Games Foundation, a program that now reaches thousands of children living in the inner cities of our nation's largest metropolitan areas.

In 1995, the American College of Sports Medicine and the Centers for Disease Control and Prevention released important recommendations for increasing the awareness of and the promotion of physical activity for all Americans. The following year, the United States government released two additional reports recommending increased physical activity. Despite these reports and recommendations, a recently released Centers for Disease Control and Prevention study concluded that the leading preventable conditions among American children today is obesity and Type 2 diabetes (the kind of diabetes that until recently was known as "adult-onset" diabetes because it tended to affect mainly obese adults). Despite these and other efforts, it appears as though we are not winning the war on sedentary lifestyles.

Until now. Walt, Dan, and Steve have taken the *ACSM Fitness Book* to a new level. Although well received in the past, this new edition includes not only the "how" but the "why" each of us should be on the road to increased physical fitness and longevity. They have included specific chapters on nutrition and weight management as well as on how to change behavior from self-destruction to health promotion. They have provided the answers to many questions most Americans have about the relationship between diet and exercise and about how to fit both into the busy American schedule. They have shown us how (and why) to make the necessary changes in our lifestyle to be healthier and to live longer. And they have dispelled myths about diet and exercise that have long been believed to be short cuts to longer lives.

With now more than 18,000 members worldwide, the scientists and practitioners of the American College of Sports Medicine have developed a real program for real people. Increase your physical activity safely and permanently. You will not regret it.

Arnold Schwarzenegger

# Preface

We are pleased to present to you the third edition of the *ACSM Fitness Book*. The book is designed for use by people interested in exercise, fitness, and health; sports professionals; other members of the health sciences community interested in and working with these disciplines; and health and fitness-oriented members of the general public. This edition updates the first and second editions to bring you the latest advice on the theory and practice of becoming fit and staying that way. This third edition has also been expanded to include separate chapters on nutrition and behavior modification. Attention to these two essential elements of becoming and staying fit has been incorporated into the entire book as well.

The ACSM, along with the Surgeon General of the United States, the Centers for Disease Control and Prevention, and the Institute of Medicine realize that a good diet is an essential part of a healthy lifestyle. We also know that effectively mobilizing motivation to change, whether in eating or exercising, is central to achieving long-term success. It happens that almost half of those who begin an exercise program drop out within three to six months. Even patients, who have a special reason for becoming regular exercisers, including those who have been diagnosed with heart disease, drop out at the same rate. This is not an accident. Too many programs for exercising or healthy eating begin and end with program specifics only, rather than, as we do in this book, with first getting the head and heart ready to make the necessary changes.

We hope that after reading chapters 2 and 3 of this book, you, your patients, and clients will not become one of the dropout statistics. Instead, we hope that the reader will be able to learn the mental skills necessary for incorporating this new and healthier lifestyle into the total pattern of living. It will then be possible to most effectively use the specific building blocks of a fitness program presented in this book that will work over the long run for the person using it.

The writers and editors of this third edition of the *ACSM Fitness Book* have had much help in putting it together. We would like to begin by thanking the editors and writers of the first and second editions. Larry Kenney was the editor of the first edition along with writers Susan Puhl, Patricia Kenney, and Arch Moore. The second edition included writers and editors Susan Puhl, Madeline Paternostro-Bayles and Barry Franklin. This third edition would not have been possible without the devotion of these teams and the success of those editions.

We would also like to thank those who reviewed drafts of the manuscript for this new edition and offered advice and criticism when it was needed. Reviewers included members of the American College of Sports Medicine Committee on Certification and Registry Boards, and Dr. Deon Thompson, Camille Civiletto, Jill Braley, Leah Long, Serena Lund, Malie Maysilles, AllisonTreby, Jeff Tamanini, Neal Pearce, Melinda Katz, Beth Dickens, Kristen Cumuze, Lynn Eubanks, Catherine Hill, and Allison Winston. Further, we would like to thank the staff of the National Office of the American College of Sports Medicine, especially D. Mark Robertson and his staff and Cathy Stewart and her staff. In addition, we would also like to thank the professionals at Human Kinetics who worked side-by-side with us to make this book come to life. They include acquisitions editor Ed McNeely, managing editor Wendy McLaughlin, assistant manager Kim Thoren, and permissions manager Toni Harte.

Finally, we would like to express our gratitude to our good friend Arnold Schwarzenegger for writing the foreword for this book. For many years, Arnold has been a steadfast crusader for improving the health of all Americans by increasing the role that physical activity plays in each of our lives.

Walt, Dan, and Steve

# CHAPTER

# 1

# An Active Lifestyle

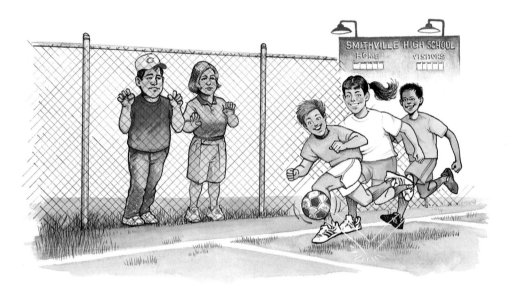

Recent polls have verified that most people believe regular exercise and good nutrition are beneficial to continued health and longevity. Those same polls also have shown that only one in five people exercises regularly. There are, of course, many reasons people do not exercise and have poor diets—not enough time, too expensive, too difficult, not the right clothes or shoes (and the list of excuses goes on and on). This book is designed to offer advice and encouragement to those who may be thinking about starting a healthier lifestyle and to those who already have an exercise program but want to learn more about it.

The decision to make exercise a regular part of your lifestyle is important, and an appropriate program can help you do it correctly. The ACSM Fitness Program is designed to help you establish and then maintain a healthy lifestyle. The activities are meant for those who may have been inactive for a few or many years and for those who are looking for additional information about diet (chapter 2), exercise (chapter 6), and the motivation to keep at it (chapter 3). Even if you consider yourself to be very unfit or if you have not exercised for many years, the ACSM Fitness Program can help you improve your health and physical fitness. Best of all, the program takes you gradually through a progressive set of exercises. You will find that exercise can be fun and does not need to be painful to be good for you.

If you have already made a commitment to improve your health through exercise and are currently exercising regularly, the fitness assessments in the ACSM Fitness Test (chapter 4) will help you determine your level of fitness and how to improve it. If the assessments indicate that you are ready for a more vigorous exercise program than the ACSM Fitness Program, the information provided in chapter 7 will help you select an appropriate and safe exercise program and motivate you to continue for a lifetime.

# Lifetime Benefits of Exercise

For many years, physicians, exercise scientists, and fitness professionals have said people should exercise regularly so they can become fit and maintain fitness. As a result, many people have come to think of exercise programs as being synonymous with vigorous physical activity, such as jogging or running. It is now known that you can achieve many health benefits from more moderate exercise, provided that you exercise often enough and long enough. Men, women, and children of any age can experience these benefits. Researchers have found that people with disabilities or chronic diseases can also benefit from regular exercise.

Health and fitness benefits increase as the amount of exercise you do increases. However, excessive amounts of exercise does not result in any additional health benefits and can prove to be detrimental. Recent research has proved that you can receive health benefits from low intensities of exercise, which may contribute to healthier living but may not necessarily improve your fitness level. The options for mild to moderate exercise are almost limitless and include such activities as walking, biking, swimming, hiking, and gardening.

# Exercising for Health

Some of the health benefits associated with regular exercise include lower risks of developing heart disease, adult-onset diabetes (type 2 diabetes), and osteoporosis. Recent scientific research also suggests that people who exercise are better able to cope with stress and are less likely to suffer from depression and anxiety. Regular exercise also helps to control weight gain (which is often associated with advancing age).

## Heart Attacks and Strokes

Regular exercise and good nutrition can have a profound risk-lowering effect on predictors associated with coronary artery disease and stroke. Regular exercise often results in modest decreases in body weight and fat content, blood pressure (in people who have mildly elevated blood pressure), blood triglyceride levels, and low-density lipoprotein (LDL) cholesterol (the

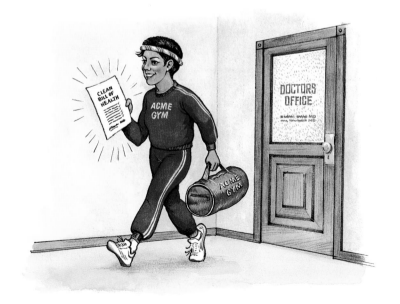

so-called "bad" cholesterol). In addition, the "good" form of cholesterol, called *high-density lipoprotein (HDL) cholesterol*, may be increased with as little as 8 to 10 miles (about 13 to 16 km) of walking per week (or the caloric equivalent of other kinds of exercise). However, for optimal improvement in blood lipids, regular aerobic exercise should be combined with a diet low in fat and cholesterol.

## Diabetes

The ability of the body to regulate the level of sugar in the blood is called *blood sugar tolerance* (or simply *glucose tolerance*). When a person's glucose tolerance declines, the concentration of sugar in the blood increases, which may lead to diabetes. Approximately one in four older adults is at risk for developing type 2 diabetes (formally known as *adult-onset* or *non-insulin-dependent diabetes*). Studies have shown that people who are physically active develop this form of diabetes less often than people who have been sedentary. Regular exercise enhances the body's ability to use insulin (a hormone that regulates the use of blood sugar) and thereby maintain normal blood sugar levels.

## Bone Density

A condition known as *osteoporosis* (a disease where the bones become more fragile over time) commonly occurs in older adults, particularly in women over the age of 50 years. As a result of the gradual loss of bone mass, even minor falls can cause broken bones, especially at the hip and at the wrist. It is well documented in the scientific and in the medical literature that weight-bearing exercise such as walking and jogging helps maintain bone density. Although improvements in bone density are generally small, it appears that regular exercise, especially for muscular strength, also helps prevent further bone loss in persons who are already affected. Such improvements may help prevent future bone fractures.

## Psychological Well-Being

People who exercise regularly have reported increased self-confidence, especially when performing physical tasks. Regular exercisers have also reported other psychological benefits such as

- an enhanced self-image and sense of well-being,
- better sleep habits,
- less depression, stress, and anxiety, and
- an improved outlook on life.

Exercise has both physiological and psychological benefits. Many adults find that their opportunities to socialize are limited, and many studies have shown that social isolation is associated with poor general health. Engaging in group activities such as dancing, golf, and water exercise not only brings people together, but also makes life more fun and interesting.

# Aerobic Fitness

Regular aerobic exercise (exercise that makes your heart and lungs work harder) increases your physical fitness, and regular, low-intensity exercise can bring about many other health benefits. Health-related fitness refers to the ability of your heart, blood vessels, lungs, and muscles to carry out daily tasks and, occasionally, unexpected physical challenges with a minimum of fatigue and discomfort. A long-term benefit of regular exercise is a reduced heart rate and blood pressure at rest and at any given level of exercise. As a result, the workload (stress) on the heart is reduced. In addition, you can do more work for a longer period of time without fatigue.

Research has shown that regular exercise also increases your ability to use oxygen, which is commonly referred to as the *maximal oxygen consumption* or *aerobic capacity* (a measure of physical fitness). Aerobic capacity is a function of how efficiently you can transport oxygen through the body and use it for the production of energy. When your aerobic capacity is high, your heart, lungs, and blood vessels are able to transport and deliver large amounts of oxygen to your body tissues. Consequently, your body can produce more energy for occupational or recreational activities, and you will not fatigue as quickly.

When your aerobic capacity improves, you will experience the following physiological changes:

- The amount of air your lungs can take in will increase because of increases in the rate and depth of your breathing.
- The amount of oxygen that moves from your lungs to your blood will increase.
- Your heart will pump more oxygen-rich blood to your muscles with each beat.
- Your muscles will be able to extract more oxygen from your blood.

A higher aerobic capacity is obviously important to a young athlete who wants to compete in a marathon, but how does it help you perform your daily activities? First, recognize that any task requires a certain amount of oxygen. Unfit people, for example, may use nearly their entire aerobic capacity to accomplish a simple activity like gardening. Although fit people will use a similar amount of oxygen for gardening, they will have more energy and be less tired because their aerobic capacity is higher. Consequently, they use a lower percentage of their maximal oxygen consumption.

# Longevity

In the United States, life expectancy at the turn of the 20th century had not yet reached 50 years. Today, life expectancy for most people living in industrialized societies is approaching 80 years, and the number of elderly people is growing at twice the rate of the rest of the population. Yet, many people often ignore exercise as a way of preparing for older age that would help ensure that the "golden years" are long and rewarding.

Low physical fitness equals a shorter life span. This equation comes from a landmark study showing that higher levels of aerobic fitness markedly decreased the risk of death from cancer, heart disease, and other chronic diseases. The men and women in the study who were the least fit had substantially higher death rates than those who were the most fit. Men who progressed from the lowest fitness level to the next-higher fitness level had the largest decrease in risk for chronic diseases. The study emphasized that the fitness level associated with the lowest mortality (death) rate could be easily achieved by most men and women if they walked briskly for 30 minutes or more every day. These and other recent findings indicate that even small increases in physical activity and fitness can have a favorable impact on longevity.

Not only does exercise contribute to longevity, but it also offers a way to reduce many of the physiological effects that are commonly assumed to be inevitable with aging. As people age, they discover that it is physically more difficult to do the activities they took for granted when they were younger, so they cut back even more. They accept rides instead of walking a short distance, and they often give up walking for pleasure. This, unfortunately, starts a vicious cycle of disuse of their body that makes them even weaker.

There is a close association between chronological aging and physical inactivity. The advancing years typically lead to the deterioration of several bodily functions, such as the ones listed in the table on the next page. The effects of regular exercise are usually positive. In recent years, scientists have shown that regular exercise may prevent some chronic diseases often associated with aging, such as heart disease, stroke, and some forms of cancer. Exercise and a sensible diet increase the quality and quantity of life.

The negative changes associated with a sedentary lifestyle often produce the stereotypical "old" person (the hunched-over, elderly woman who wears sweaters in the summer and can no longer open a jar of pickles or the man whose walk has turned into a shuffle and who is so stiff he can barely bend over to tie his shoelaces). Exercise clearly reduces or prevents many of these adverse effects of aging. The protective and perhaps restorative potential of regular physical activity is a matter of critical importance to billions of people who are moving toward older age. For example, consider the age-related deterioration in our ability to take in and use oxygen. After people reach 20 years of age, without the benefit of regular exercise their aerobic capacity (a key indicator of our capacity to produce energy) typically decreases by about one percent per year.

## Effects of Aging and Exercise on the Body and Its Functions

| Variable | Effect of aging | Effect of exercise |
| --- | --- | --- |
| Aerobic fitness | negative | positive |
| Heart function | negative | positive |
| Blood pressure | negative | positive |
| Strength | negative | positive |
| Resting metabolism | negative | positive |
| Insulin activity | negative | positive |
| Blood fats | negative | positive |
| Bone density | negative | positive |
| Temperature regulation | negative | positive |
| Joint mobility | negative | positive |
| Psychological well-being | negative | positive |
| Senses* | negative | positive |
| Memory | negative | positive |

*Hearing, eyesight, taste, smell

Because an exercise program will usually increase this variable by about 20 percent, the physically active 60-year-old can achieve the same fitness level as the inactive 40-year-old. In other words, regular exercise can lead to a 20-year functional rejuvenation. The saying "use it or lose it" seems particularly applicable when it comes to slowing the aging process. To further illustrate this point, if the 20-year rejuvenation continues, the shuffling 80-year-old could become the fast-walking 60-year-old who is still playing golf!

# Physical Activity for All

An expert panel commissioned by the Centers for Disease Control and Prevention, the U.S. Surgeon General, and the American College of Sports Medicine reviewed the research on the health benefits of regular physical activity. The recommendations of the panel were expressed in this concise public health message:

*"Every adult should accumulate 30 minutes or more of moderate-intensity physical activity on most, preferably all, days of the week."*

Whether you are interested in improving overall health, increasing aerobic fitness, or slowing the aging process, this is great advice.

# What Is Fitness?

Earlier in this chapter, health-related physical fitness was described as the ability of your heart, blood vessels, lungs, and muscles to carry out daily tasks and occasional, unexpected physical challenges with a minimum of fatigue and discomfort. Stated another way, it is having the reserve to do all that you want to do—and more.

Becoming fit does not require high-intensity physical activity, monotonous workouts, or even an expensive health club membership (although this is sometimes motivational, as you will read in a later chapter). To become physically fit, you simply need a regular program of exercise and healthy nutrition (see chapter 2). To become healthy and to sustain good health, a regular program of diet and exercise is a big step in the right direction.

You need to understand, though, that physical fitness is a lifetime pursuit. A program that lasts only 10 or 12 weeks will not bring about a lifetime of fitness benefits. Unfortunately, if you stop exercising, your fitness gains may be lost over a short period.

Health-related physical fitness actually has four components:

 *Aerobic fitness* is the body's ability to take in and use oxygen to produce energy.

 *Muscular fitness* is the strength and endurance of your muscles.

 *Flexibility* is the ability to bend joints and stretch muscles through a full range of motion.

 *Body composition* is the amount of fat tissue relative to other tissue in your body.

Because fitness has four different components, the *ACSM Fitness Book* provides you with a physical conditioning program that includes exercises to improve your fitness in all areas. The book also offers advice on maintaining a good diet and how to stay mentally fit. All these components are important to staying healthy for a lifetime.

# Aerobic Fitness

The ACSM Fitness Program uses walking as an example of how to improve aerobic fitness. Walking offers easily tolerated exercise intensity and causes fewer musculoskeletal and orthopedic problems of the lower extremities than jogging or running. It is also an activity that requires no special equipment other than a pair of well-fitted athletic shoes. Other effective exercises that use large muscle groups can also improve your aerobic fitness. Such activities include stationary or outdoor bicycling, rowing, swimming, skating, stair climbing, hiking, and simulated or real cross-country skiing.

# Muscular Fitness

Muscular fitness is essential to most of your daily tasks, whether it is lifting a child or pushing a lawnmower. Manipulating your body and the objects around you requires that you have enough strength to move the things you want to move and enough endurance to hold the items or the position successfully. The ACSM Fitness Program uses a variety of exercises to improve both the strength and endurance of the major muscles of your upper and lower body.

## Flexibility

All movements of muscles and joints require some degree of flexibility. Joints and muscles that are not flexible limit movement and increase the risk of pain and even injury. When you improve your flexibility, you help prevent strains and other problems, such as back pain (which affects nearly half of the adult population). Regular stretching exercises will help increase your flexibility. The ACSM Fitness Program includes stretching exercises for all the major joints of the body.

## Body Composition

Your body composition is based not on how much you weigh, but rather on how much of your weight is fat and how much is considered lean (including muscles, bones, and organs). Excessive body fat can cause musculoskeletal problems and increase your risk of heart disease, stroke, diabetes, and high blood pressure. On the other end of the spectrum, too little fat is associated with other medical conditions. You can have a heavy, athletic physique and have little body fat, or be thin but have poor muscle development and relatively more fat. The ACSM Fitness Program suggests that regular exercise, such as walking or other aerobic activities, along with muscular fitness exercises, will favorably modify body composition.

# Three Simple Steps to Fitness

The ACSM Fitness Program is designed to help you take the guesswork out of planning a safe, effective exercise routine to enhance all areas of physical fitness. It takes you through a simple three-step approach to developing and maintaining fitness:

1. Find out where you are.
2. Design a program to achieve your goals—and stick with achieving them.
3. Check your progress.

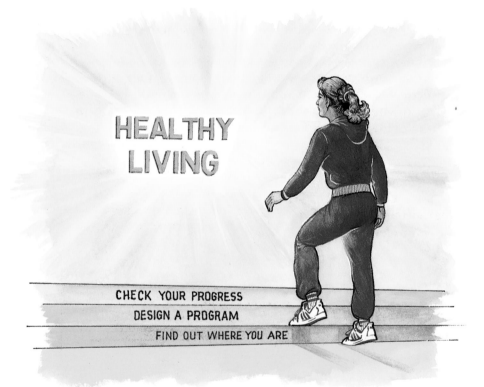

## Step 1. Baseline Assessment

A little later in this chapter and in chapter 3, you will be taught how to set appropriate goals. To help you reach your goals, it is important to know your current fitness status. Otherwise, you might choose an exercise program that is too difficult (or too easy) for you. Chapter 4 presents a simple four-part test (the ACSM Fitness Test) to help determine your level in each of the four components of physical fitness just described.

# Step 2. Design a Program to Achieve Your Goals

Your personal ACSM Fitness Program is based on your scores in each of the four fitness components. You will use the scores to build your exercise program (which will be color-coded in the rest of the book, so you can easily follow the steps). You may find, for example, that your test results indicate you are at a higher level in the aerobic fitness component than in the flexibility component. The ACSM Fitness Program allows you to choose the exercises that correspond to your fitness level for each of these important components. In that way, you can be sure that the exercises are neither too difficult nor too easy in any area of fitness development.

Chapter 6 will provide an easy-to-follow, day-by-day exercise schedule for each level in the four components of physical fitness. Each level of the program takes you through six weeks of activities. The daily schedule includes specific exercises for you to complete. You will start at the appropriate level for each fitness component and continue until you successfully complete the entire program. When you finish one level of the program, you will be instructed on how to proceed to the next level. You will continue to progress until you have completed all levels of the program or until you have reached your fitness goals. Your fitness will continue to improve in a safe and enjoyable manner.

# Step 3. Check Your Progress

Keeping track of your progress in your ACSM Fitness Program is like checking the highway signs on a cross-country trip: It helps you know exactly where you are. In chapter 6, you will find record sheets for tracking your progress. Keeping records takes only a few seconds, but it will be very important to your total program. It takes the guesswork out of trying to remember what you did and how you felt each time you exercised. As you work through the program, you will also want to periodically review the goals you have set for yourself. When you achieve a goal, reward yourself in some way—then set a new goal. It is easier to stay with your exercise program when you can see the progress you have made.

# You Can Do It!

Now you are motivated to begin a program to improve your health and fitness, help you live longer, and increase the quality of your life. What will be the secret of your success? In a word, persistence! Many people exercise for a while, but the results seem to come too slowly, so they stop and go looking for something easier. What they do not realize is that if they had hung on just a little bit longer, they could have reached their goals and reaped the rewards of healthful living.

Unfortunately, when it comes to a lifestyle change such as getting regular exercise, many people think that it is an all-or-nothing proposition. Achieving good health and physical fitness is similar to running a marathon, not sprinting (see chapter 3). It is what you do over the long term that really counts. Do not worry about one particular point in the race when you may not have performed as well as you had hoped. All too often, people give up their exercise programs because they have failed to follow them perfectly. They mistakenly reason that all is lost, and they go back to their old ways. Remember, the key word is *persistence.*

By reading this book, you have taken a significant step to making regular exercise part of your life. It is important to realize that the favorable impact on health and fitness that results from a program of exercise occurs only when you stick with the program. While most people can be encouraged to begin a good exercise program, fewer than half the people who start one actually stay with it. Some people become bored with exercise or don't have the commitment to stick with a program. It might be difficult for them to find a convenient time to exercise, or they become frustrated because they are not seeing the results of their program as quickly as they would like. When it comes to sustaining interest and enthusiasm, these negative variables can really derail a program.

To help yourself maintain your motivation to sustain a regular exercise commitment, acknowledge that it may compete with other valued interests and responsibilities of your daily life. It should become, however, another commitment of your daily (and now healthy) lifestyle. Here are several things you can do, beyond relying on mere willpower, to maintain and to increase your motivation.

• **Learn all you can about the benefits of exercise.** If you thoroughly understand the benefits that can be achieved by following a regular exercise program, you will be more inclined to stick with it. Good instruction provided by qualified exercise professionals, such as those certified by the American College of Sports Medicine, will give you the knowledge to develop an exercise program that is both safe and effective.

• **Minimize your chance of injury by choosing mild to moderate exercise.** Too often beginning exercisers become discouraged because their muscles are sore or they have become injured from working out too vigorously or from stepping up the pace too quickly. For the beginner, an excessive exercise frequency (more than five workouts per week), duration (more than 45 minutes per session), or intensity (always working at hard to very hard effort) offers little additional gain in fitness but disproportionately increases the chance for injury. A starter program may include just 20 to 30 minutes of exercise every other day at a comfortable intensity (fairly light to somewhat intense). Warm up and cool down adequately, and be sure to wear proper

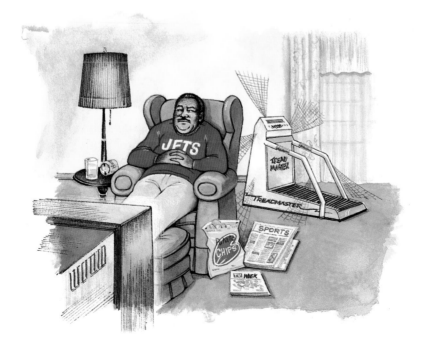

shoes and socks. Once you have become accustomed to the activity, then increase the duration or frequency first before increasing the intensity. A long-term goal should be to accumulate 30 minutes or more of moderately intensive physical activity on most days of the week.

- **Establish short-term goals.** Goal setting should be viewed much like climbing a ladder, with emphasis placed on reasonable distances between the rungs. Refer back to the section titled "Benefits of Exercise," then set goals that relate to those benefits that are most important to you. As you set your goals, follow these guidelines:

a. Make your goals challenging, but realistic. For example, if it presently takes you 18 minutes to walk a mile, an appropriate beginning goal would be to walk a mile in 15 minutes rather than in 11 minutes.

b. Set specific, not general, goals. Rather than setting a goal "to improve muscular strength," aim to increase the number of push-ups you can do at one time from 10 to 15.

c. Set short-term goals. Set goals that you can reach within a time period that is short enough to keep you motivated. Rather than setting a goal of losing 35 pounds this year, set one to lose 3 pounds this month.

Take a few minutes to think about your personal fitness goals. After you have identified several, write them down in the first section of the chart below. As you reach your goals, you can set new ones, recording them in a second section, a third section, and then more sections. As you continue with your exercise program, your list will help remind you how much you have achieved.

| Date | Personal Fitness Goals |
|---|---|
| | 1. |
| | 2. |
| | 3. |

- **Consider joining a group or exercising with a friend.** Commitments made, as part of a group, tend to be stronger than those made independently. The stimulus of the group often provides the incentive to continue during periods of flagging interest. Better long-term adherence has been reported in programs that incorporate group dynamics as compared with those in which one exercises alone.

- **Do activities you enjoy.** When exercise is fun or pleasurable, it will help you maintain motivation. You should select activities that you would look forward to, not dread.

- **Complete a fitness assessment periodically to check your progress.** Take a fitness test before you start your exercise program, and at regular intervals, to assess your response to the exercise program. Favorable changes in these evaluations can serve as powerful motivators that produce renewed interest and dedication. Chapter 4 explains how to complete the ACSM Fitness Test.

- **Record your exercise achievements on a progress chart.** Research shows the importance of immediate positive feedback on the reinforcement of health-related behaviors. A progress chart that allows you to record your daily exercise achievements can help with this objective. In chapter 6, you will find record sheets for tracking your progress.

- **No time? Consider multiple short bouts of exercise.** Recent studies suggest that multiple short bouts of physical exercise yield improvements in fitness similar to those yielded by single long bouts, provided that the total amount of time spent exercising is comparable. For many persons, several short bouts of exercise may fit better into a busy schedule than a single long bout. If you cannot find 30 minutes a day to exercise, consider two 15-minute or three 10-minute sessions spread throughout the day.

- **Establish a schedule.** Make exercise an important part of your day—make it a habit. Early morning workouts may make exercise a higher priority. You might be tempted to cancel late afternoon or evening workouts because of fatigue or unscheduled meetings or delays. Try this trick to help motivate you to stick with your exercise program: Buy a large glass jar and display it prominently in your home. Put a coin in the jar for each day you reasonably follow your exercise plan. If you fail to exercise for a scheduled exercise day, take out a coin (or even two), but do not empty out all the precious coins that you have saved to that point. When the jar is full, go out and buy yourself something special. You will be well on your way to the health and fitness goals that you desire.

We hope you see how easy it will be for you to use this book and to participate in the ACSM Fitness Program. We have done the planning for you, so you can put all your energy into improving your fitness.

CHAPTER

# 2

# Nutrition, Physical Activity, and Health

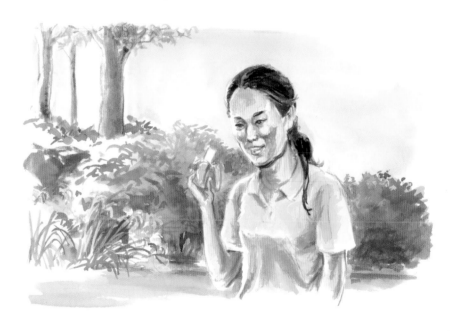

**N**utrition, physical activity, and health are strongly connected. Although this book often focuses on the specifics of each area independently, it is impossible to be physically active or fit without meeting one's nutritional needs; and being physically active and physically fit alters one's nutritional requirements. Despite the interdependence of physical activity and nutrition, people often try to satisfy their need for healthful exercise and good nutrition as if the two were not connected—and this is a mistake. Your food intake should match your dynamics of physical activity because the two are so closely related.

You must consider several things in the development of an optimal marriage between physical activity and nutrition. The most critical is this: Physical activity increases the rate at which energy (that is, calories) is burned, and this creates a higher caloric requirement (the use of the words *caloric*, *calorie*, and *calories* refers to the commonly used measuring unit for energy in human nutrition, which is equivalent to *kilocalorie* and *kcal*). Therefore, the higher your intensity of physical activity, the greater your need for muscular fuel (i.e., calories). The fuel used by working muscles must be drawn from fuel reserves, which are stored in muscles in varying degrees, or must be consumed during the activity so that the fuel can be delivered directly to working muscles. As more fuel is burned, there is also an increased need for certain other nutrients, such as vitamins, minerals, and fluid. Of course, the reverse is also true: Less physical activity requires a lower need for fuel, certain nutrients, and fluid. Too often, people overcompensate for their energy needs. In the United States alone, over 50 percent of the population is now considered overweight or obese. This is a very scary statistic! Here is your goal: Learn how to balance your caloric and nutrient needs with physical activity to achieve a state of optimal health.

# The Exercise–Energy Relationship

The relationship between exercise and energy is simple: For weight maintenance, caloric intake must equal caloric expenditure. To lose weight, you must have a caloric intake that is less than caloric expenditure. For weight gain, caloric intake must be greater than caloric expenditure. Physical activity increases the demand for energy, so you must learn how much food to consume to satisfy your need for calories and nutrients.

## Timing of Meals

You cannot run your car when the gas tank is empty, and you cannot make your muscles run on empty either. *When* and *how often* you eat during the day are just as important to consider as how much you eat over the course of a day. People often think about total calories consumed during the day but rarely consider how best to deliver those calories.

Consider the following example: You are driving a car from New York City to Miami and planning how best to fuel your automobile. You are considering three possible options:

1. Wait until you arrive in Miami, and then give your car all the fuel it needed for the trip.

2. Give the car all the fuel it needs before you leave New York City. (The car has to figure out where and how to store all this fuel.)

3. Fill up your car with fuel before you leave New York City, and stop every 300 miles (483 km) to refill the tank.

It is obvious that options 1 and 2 are not possible and not logical. Yet, despite the fact that option 3 is clearly the most logical way to fuel the car, people typically use either option 1 or 2 to fuel themselves during the day. Exercisers are well known for their predisposition to "back load" their food or fuel intake. That is, they do not eat enough to support their physical activity, but after the physical activity and other daily activities are over, they eat a large meal at the end of the day to take in the calories they

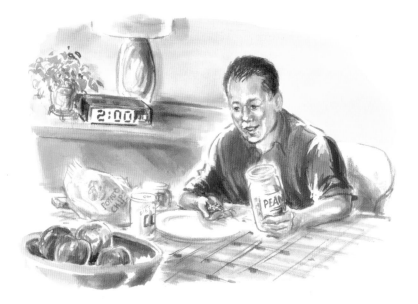

needed earlier. The opposite is also true: Many people who exercise try to consume a huge amount of food several hours before an exercise bout or competition, but the level of energy consumed far exceeds the body's capacity to optimally process that amount of energy at one time. The result is an excess of fat storage. Options 1 and 2 are strategies that do not work for cars, and these strategies do not work for humans, either.

Everyone has a different metabolism, resulting in a slightly different rate of caloric "burn." Despite these subtle differences, the following guide will provide you with a general estimate of how much energy you need over a 24-hour period.

## Estimating Caloric Needs

When calculating the number of calories you need to consume to function optimally on a day-to-day basis, remember to round to the nearest whole number. Follow the instructions to find your own energy requirements based on your personal statistics.

1. Take your weight in pounds and divide by 2.2 to calculate your weight in kilograms:

    Example for a 160-pound male:
    160 pounds ÷ 2.2 = 72.7 kilograms, or 73 kilograms

2. Weight in kilograms represents the approximate number of calories this 160-pound (73-kilogram) male requires to maintain his weight during 1 hour of rest. Multiply this number by 24 to obtain the approximate number of calories this person requires in a day (24 hours):

    73 kilograms × 24 hours = 1,752 calories per day at rest

3. To calculate the calories required for activity, use the information found in the following chart. For instance, if the male in our example were moderately active, you would multiply the calories per day at rest by a number between .65 and .80:

    1,752 calories at rest × .70 (moderate activity factor) = 1,226.4, or 1,226 activity calories

4. Now add the calories per day at rest to the activity calories to obtain the approximate daily caloric requirement:

1,752 calories at rest + 1,226 activity calories = 2,978 calories per day (for this example)

Infrequent eating patterns force people to consume more at each meal to satisfy their need for energy, whereas more frequent eating patterns allow a smaller consumption during each meal. For instance, a long-distance runner consuming an 1,800-calorie high-carbohydrate meal the evening before a race is likely to easily exceed his or her carbohydrate storage capacity. The result is that a significant proportion of this meal is stored as fat, making it unavailable as energy in the form of carbohydrate. So try to spread your calories throughout the day—as in the example with the car. This way you'll have the energy you need when you need it and you won't be bogged down with extra storage of fat. The following table shows the adjustment factors for various activity levels in men and women when calculating total daily caloric needs.

| Activity Levels in Men and Women | | |
|---|---|---|
| Activity Level | Male | Female |
| **Sedentary** (Spends almost no time walking or doing any physical work; is sleeping, sitting or reclining most of the day) | .25 to .40 | .25 to .35 |
| **Light** (Spends a small amount of time each day walking or doing other seated activities) | .50 to .70 | .40 to .60 |
| **Moderate** (Spends some time in the day in physical work of moderate intensity, such as brisk walks, and garden work.) | .65 to .80 | .50 to .70 |
| **Heavy** (Spends an important portion of the day in heavy physical activity or work.) | .90 to 1.20 | .80 to 1.00 |
| **Extremely Heavy** (Spends a large portion of the day in heavy, exhaustive physical activity or work.) | 1.30 to 1.45 | 1.10 to 1.30 |

# Deciding What and How Much Energy You Need

The general recommendation for achieving an optimum state of health is to consume the majority of energy in the form of carbohydrates (particularly complex carbohydrates such as whole grain foods and fresh fruits and vegetables), a smaller amount of energy from protein, and a small to moderate amount of fat. How much and what kinds of food should you eat? Let's start with the main components—carbohydrates, proteins, and fat.

## Carbohydrates

Carbohydrates can be either simple or complex. Common simple carbohydrates include glucose, fructose, and sucrose; these *sugars* are typically associated with sweet foods and ripe fruits such as apples, bananas, peaches, pears, and berries. Complex carbohydrates are either digestible (starches) or indigestible (fiber). Digestible complex carbohydrates are ultimately digested to the simple carbohydrate called *glucose*. The ultimate fuel for muscles is glucose, which is stored in the body as glycogen. However, complex carbohydrate foods usually carry with them other nutrients, such as the B vitamins, which are necessary for muscles to get energy from the foods we have eaten. Foods rich in simple carbohydrates (pure sugars such as table sugar, honey, or the sugar found in soft drinks), on the other hand, do provide energy but may not contain other required nutrients. Therefore, it is generally recom-

### Low Carb, High Protein, High Fat—Okay?

Recently, much attention has been given to low-carbohydrate diets, particularly as weight-loss regimens. However, focusing on either fats or proteins as the main sources of energy is counterproductive both for good health and for optimum exercise performance. In addition, the higher fat intakes associated with these diets increase the risks for heart disease and may increase the risks for certain cancers. When low-carbohydrate diets successfully produce weight loss, it is typically because of a loss of body water and a reduction in total caloric intake rather than because of the reduction in *carbohydrate* intake.

mended that people who exercise consume no less than 60 percent of their total calories from carbohydrates and no more than 10 percent of these calories in the form of simple carbohydrates (sugars and refined grains). Good sources of carbohydrates include pasta, bread, cereal, legumes (beans), fruits, and vegetables.

## Protein

Protein makes up about 45 percent of the human body and is an essential part of blood, muscles, bone, hormones, antibodies, and enzymes. Protein is an important constituent of the diet, but the amount of protein we actually need for activity and health is considerably less than many people think.

Muscle is approximately 70 percent water and only about 20 percent protein. Therefore, increasing muscle mass requires extra water, additional calories in the form of carbohydrates (to maintain the energy needs of that extra muscle), and a little extra protein. In fact, for someone increasing muscle mass at an extraordinarily high rate of 1 kilogram per week (2.2 pounds of extra muscle per week), only 4 extra ounces (113.4 grams) of meat per day would be needed in the diet. Why are so many people convinced that increasing protein intake helps them do physical work? The most likely reason is that the extra protein consumed is helping them meet total caloric requirements.

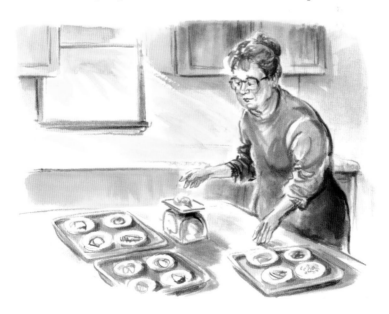

Good sources of protein include meat, poultry, fish, and eggs. However, vegetarians can obtain adequate protein by combining nonmeat items. For instance, combining legumes (beans) and whole grains (rice or corn) creates a protein combination of high quality. However, animal proteins provide numerous other nutrients (including iron and zinc) that are more difficult to obtain elsewhere unless the diet is very carefully planned.

Inadequate protein intake may, however, be a concern for some people. Children have higher protein requirements than adults because their growth increases the requirement for protein. A child who is physically active would have an even higher protein requirement. Many young people involved in sports have difficulty consuming enough total energy to satisfy the combined needs of growth and physical activity; and when total energy intake is inadequate, protein intake may also be inadequate. Vegetarians and people who are on weight-loss diets may also be putting themselves at risk of having inadequate protein intakes. Regardless of need, however, protein requirements are always relatively small compared to the need for carbohydrates. For instance, a 150-pound (68-kilogram) man who exercises frequently would have a protein requirement of 136 grams of protein per day (this is 544 calories per day from protein). Compare this to the approximately 680 grams of carbohydrates the same person would require (this is 2,720 calories per day from carbohydrates).

## Fat

Despite what many consumers think, fat is an important energy source that provides us with the essential fatty acids and carries fat-soluble vitamins (vitamins A, D, E, and K). In general, however, people eat more fat than is desirable for health or is necessary for physical activity. Americans typically consume foods that provide well over 35 percent of total calories from fat, and surveys of people who exercise regularly indicate that their average fat intake is only slightly lower. Physically active people should strive to have a fat intake that does not exceed 25 percent of total calories. To achieve this goal, it is important to know what foods are high in fat and to develop strategies to make it easier to reduce fat intake.

Fats are metabolized during exercise, but it takes time and aerobic training to become an efficient fat "burner." Besides being a highly concentrated source of energy, excess dietary fat is very efficiently and easily converted to stored body fat. Therefore, a combination of frequent exercise and lower dietary fat are both needed to assure a good body fat level. The good news is you do not have to totally eliminate fat from your diet.

Here are some simple rules that will help lower your fat intake:

1. Avoid fried foods by consuming the nonfried equivalent (baked chicken instead of fried chicken, broiled fish instead of fried fish, baked potato instead of French-fried potatoes).

2. Avoid high-fat dairy products by consuming skim or low-fat dairy products (more than 40 percent of the calories from whole milk comes from fat and more than 30 percent of the calories from 2 percent milk comes from fat. Try to consume skim milk or 1 percent milk and milk products).

3. Avoid visible fats such as butter, margarine, and the fat on meats. (If you are accustomed to having toast with butter and jam in the morning, have the toast and jam but skip the butter.)

4. Avoid prepared and processed meats, such as hot dogs, bologna, and salami, which are usually very high in fat, by consuming lean roast beef, chicken breast (without skin), and turkey breast (without skin).

5. Avoid pre-packaged convenience foods, particularly those described as "crispy"; these tend to be extremely high in fat.

# Weight and Body Composition Goals

How much energy you should consume and how you distribute the energy substrates (proteins, carbohydrates, and fats) has much to do with your weight and body composition goals. The generally accepted recommendation is to reduce daily caloric intakes by 500 calories to achieve a 1-pound-per-week (or 0.45-kilogram-per-week) weight loss. Because most people like to eat, the easiest way to lower caloric intake is to reduce fat intake and replace the fatty foods with more complex carbohydrates (fruits, vegetables, whole grains, legumes). This will give you the energy you need to exercise and function while avoiding excess stored fat. Use the following table as a general guide.

## Exercise and Eating Strategies for Reducing Obesity

| Exercise | Gradually increase the amount and intensity of exercise. <br> · Focus on activities that are enjoyed. <br> · Focus on activities that move the body over a distance. <br> · Exercise with friends or peers who will encourage a regular exercise schedule. <br> · Become involved in activities that can be pursued for a lifetime. |
|---|---|
| Nutrition | · Avoid severe caloric restriction. <br> · Eat small meals frequently to avoid severe hunger. <br> · Avoid fad diets, supplements, and drugs. <br> · Avoid dehydration as a weight-loss strategy. <br> · Consume adequate carbohydrate, protein, and other nutrients, but try to lower fat intake to no more than 15 to 25% of total calories. <br> · To lose weight you must be in a negative caloric balance, but you should not exceed a daily caloric deficit of 500 calories. This will lead to a consistent weight loss of approximately 1 lb (0.45 kg) per week. While this may not sound like much, if consistently pursued, the amount of such a weight loss would be more than 50 lb (23 kg) in one year. |

Reprinted, by permission, from 2001, "ACSM position paper on the appropriate intervention strategies for weight loss and prevention of weight gain for adults," *MSSE* 33 (12) 2145-2156.

People often get hungry between meals. When that happens they may consume high-fat convenience foods as between-meal snacks because they fail to plan for the inevitable hunger that will occur. If you allow yourself to get excessively hungry, you will inevitably eat too much when you finally have a chance to eat, making it difficult to achieve a moderate energy intake reduction. To avoid excessive hunger, be prepared to have a small snack between meals. This snack should be between 150 to 250 calories of complex carbohydrates, such as fruit(s), whole grain products (for instance, two slices of whole-wheat toast), raw or cooked vegetables, or pre-packaged whole-grain energy bars. Consider preparing your mid-morning and mid-afternoon snacks to take with you before you leave the house in the morning, so you will never have to wonder what you will eat for your between-meal snack. The nutritional strategies and exercise recommendations presented in this book will help guide you toward a more ideal body weight and better overall health.

# Vitamins, Minerals, and Supplements

All vitamins and minerals in human nutrition are equally important. And, despite what you may hear in the media, it appears that some people are at risk for a deficiency of only a *few* vitamins and minerals, including iron, calcium, and folic acid. Do not be misled into thinking that only these nutrients are important, however. Nutrients work together, so missing any nutrient or having too much of another may alter your nutritional balance to such a degree that you will have problems achieving optimal health and fitness. A good way to think about your vitamin and mineral needs is this: All cells in your body have a requirement for a certain array of vitamins and minerals, in varying quantities. Your job is to assure that these cells are exposed to what they need. Providing too little of a given vitamin or mineral may cause the cell to malfunction, and providing too much will cause the cell to expend extra energy to get rid of the excess. The best strategy for ensuring that you are exposed to a wide spectrum of vitamins and minerals is to eat a wide variety of foods and in that way avoid consuming the same few foods all the time.

## B Vitamins

B vitamins work together in processing the energy you consume. They are, therefore, very important to people who exercise. However, taking supplements, in the absence of a known deficiency, does *not* improve athletic potential, and may even introduce harmful side effects. Therefore, a balanced diet is the best approach to making certain you get enough of the B vitamins (review the following table).

Because these vitamins are linked to physical activity, inadequate intake of B vitamins will result in easy fatigue and poor physical performance. However, because physically active people typically consume more food, they also consume more of these vitamins in the process. Therefore, B vitamin deficiencies are

## Food Sources of B Vitamins

| Vitamin | Food Sources |
| --- | --- |
| Thiamin ($B_1$) | Liver, pork, lean meats, wheat germ, whole grains, enriched breads, and cereals |
| Riboflavin ($B_2$) | Milk and milk products, liver, enriched breads, and cereals |
| Niacin | Liver, poultry, fish, peanut butter |
| Pyridoxine ($B_6$) | Liver, herring and salmon, wheat germ and whole grains, lean meats |
| Folic Acid | Liver, wheat bran, whole grains, spinach and other green leafy vegetables, legumes, orange juice |
| Vitamin $B_{12}$ | Foods of animal origin, specially prepared fermented yeasts, and fortified soy products |
| Biotin | Egg Yolk, liver, and legumes |
| Pantothenic Acid | Eggs, liver, wheat bran, peanuts, legumes, lean meats, spinach, and other vegetables |

most likely to occur in people who are purposefully reducing food intake to lower weight or in people on monotonous intakes (i.e., who continuously eat the same few foods without varying food intake.)

# Vitamin C

Everyone has heard of the health benefits of vitamin C, but what does it really do? Vitamin C helps the body absorb iron, resist infection, and metabolize food. Vitamin C is associated with fresh foods, including fruits, fruit juices, bean sprouts, and vegetables. Because of this, vitamin C intake is often considered a marker for the quality of a person's diet. An adequate intake (several servings each day) of fresh fruits and vegetables is a certain way to consume enough vitamin C. Some great sources of vitamin C include strawberries, citrus fruits (such as oranges and grapefruits), tomatoes, bean sprouts, and cherries.

# Calcium

Calcium is necessary for strong bones. It makes sense that the more physical stress you put on your bones, the stronger your bones will need to be, but many people who exercise have a calcium intake that is far less than the recommended amount. Bones consist of living cells that are constantly changing (just like all other cells in the body). Providing enough calcium helps to ensure that the bone cells will change in a positive direction. In addition to adding strength to bones, calcium has several other important functions, including involvement in nerve impulse transmission, muscle contraction, blood clotting, acid–base balance (pH control), and blood pressure control. Inadequate calcium intake can increase the risk of stress fractures, and inadequate intake during childhood and adolescence may increase the risk of early osteoporosis (bone disease) later in life.

The intake goal for calcium should be between 800 and 1,500 milligrams per day. Because one cup of milk provides approximately 300 milligrams of calcium, an equivalent of three to five cups of milk (or foods containing the same concentration of calcium, such as calcium-fortified orange juice) should be consumed daily (see the following table). If you are certain the foods you consume will not provide you with enough calcium, then taking a 250- to 500-milligram supplement of calcium daily (e.g., calcium carbonate, calcium lactate, or calcium citrate) is a good strategy.

# Iron

Iron deficiency is one of the most common nutrient deficiencies and particularly affects adolescent girls and women in their childbearing years. Vegetarians are also at a higher risk of iron deficiency because red meat (not consumed by vegetarians) is one of the best sources of dietary iron. This does not mean that all females, children undergoing fast growth, and vegetarians will suffer from iron deficiency. It just means that these groups must be especially careful that they consume an adequate amount of iron in the foods they consume. Getting enough iron in your diet is important: An iron deficiency may inhibit your ability to exercise because iron is involved in carrying oxygen to cells and in removing carbon dioxide from them. Some physically active people may be at risk for iron deficiency because of poor iron intake, poor iron absorption, loss of iron in sweat, blood loss in the GI tract, or an increased rate of red blood cell breakdown.

## Calcium Content of Foods

**The following foods contain about the same amount of calcium (297mg) as 8 oz (1 cup) of milk**

| | |
|---|---|
| Cheddar cheese | 1.5 oz |
| Cottage cheese | 2 cups |
| Yogurt | 1 cup |
| Processed cheese | 1.5 slices |
| Ice cream | 1.5 cups |
| Ice milk | 1.5 cups |
| Tofu | 8 oz. |
| Broccoli | 2 cups |
| Collard greens | 1 cup |
| Turnip greens | 1 cup |
| Mustard greens | 1.5 cups |
| Salmon | 4 oz. |
| Sardines | 2.5 oz. |
| Orange juice with calcium | 1 cup |

## Strategies for Reducing Iron Deficiency Risk

- Consume lean cuts of meat (dark poultry or red meat) three to four times per week.
- Consume enriched grains and cereals (such as breads and pastas).
- Consume foods containing vitamin C (such as fruits and fruit juices) with grains and vegetables. The vitamin C enhances iron absorption from these foods.

- Consume tea, coffee, and all-bran products in moderation. These foods contain substances that may inhibit iron absorption.
- Women of childbearing age may require a low-level supplement of iron to ensure adequate intake (consult your physician).

# Ergogenic Aids

*Ergogenic aids* are substances that enhance the ability of a person to do physical work, either through improvements in power or enhanced endurance. Athletes often take ergogenic aids because they are advertised as giving them a competitive advantage, either by helping them train harder and longer or by improving performance on the day of competition. There are two ergogenic aids that have been clearly established as improving a person's ability to do physical work and improve athletic performance: carbohydrates and water. With the exception of these, there is very little evidence to suggest that other substances frequently touted as having an "ergogenic effect" actually do anything to improve athletic performance.

When ergogenic aids do work, it is usually because they help a person meet energy or nutritional requirements that are a result of less than ideal eating behaviors. It is clearly healthier and less costly to eat better foods than to rely on substances that are often of unknown origin, unknown quality, and that remain untested for effectiveness or safety. In addition, the International Olympic Committee, International Paralympic Committee, the National Collegiate Athletic Association, the United States Olympic Committee, and other national sports governing bodies ban many ergogenic aids, because they have not been adequately tested for safety or effectiveness. If you are confronted with a decision on whether to take a pill or capsule to improve your ability to exercise, you should seriously consider doing the right thing: Eat small frequent meals that are high in complex carbohydrates and include plenty of fluids to maintain a desirable energized state, and avoid other ergogenic aids that are likely to be expensive and inadequately tested.

# Water, Water, Water!

Water is essential for human life. It is needed to transport nutrients to cells and to remove toxic metabolic by-products away from cells. The evaporation of water cools the body and helps to maintain a constant body temperature. Water is also the most critical single nutrient needed to ensure that a person can safely sustain physical activity. Because heat production is increased with *all* forms of exercise, it is necessary for physically active people to maintain water balance so this excess heat can be dissipated through the production of sweat. With the evaporation of sweat, heat is lost from the blood that circulates near the skin. The rate of sweat loss varies between people and with the outside temperature, but it is common to see water losses of up to three liters (more than six quarts!) per hour in fit people who exercise in hot and humid environments.

## Dehydration

Dehydration occurs when fluid losses are greater than 1 percent of body weight, and athletic ability is impaired with a 2 percent loss of body weight. This means a person weighing 100 pounds (or 45 kilograms) who loses 2 pounds (.9 kilograms) during exercise may no longer be performing up to her trained ability because of the excessive water loss. Be aware that water loss that represents 6 percent of body weight may occur after two hours of exercise in high heat. Typical symptoms of inadequate fluid intake during exercise include thirst, fatigue, loss of coordination, mental confusion, irritability, dry skin, elevated body temperature, and reduced urine output.

Heat stroke (caused by severe heat injury and inadequate hydration) has a death rate of 80 percent! To be sure you are getting enough water to meet your body's needs, drink at least eight glasses of fluids on any normal day and more than that on days with high temperatures and humidity. If you are exercising, be sure to drink at least one glass of fluid before *and* after exercise and every 10 to 15 minutes during exercise to make sure you replenish all fluids lost to sweat. Do not substitute water with soda, coffee, or tea. These beverages contain caffeine that acts as a diuretic and may reduce the amount of water in your body.

## Guidelines for Proper Hydration

1. Consume a nutritionally balanced diet and drink adequate fluids during the 24-hour period before an event, especially during the period that includes the meal prior to exercise, to promote proper hydration before exercise or competition.

2. Drink about one half-liter (about 17 ounces) of fluid about two hours before exercise to promote adequate hydration and to allow time for excretion of excess ingested water.

3. During exercise, start drinking early and at regular intervals to consume fluids at a rate sufficient enough to replace all the water lost through sweating (body weight loss), or consume the maximal amount that can be tolerated.

4. Keep fluids cooler than ambient temperature (between 15 and 22 degrees Celsius [59 and 72 degrees Fahrenheit]) and try flavored sport drinks to enhance palatability and promote fluid replacement. Fluids should be readily available and served in containers that allow adequate volumes to be ingested with ease and with minimal interruption of exercise.

5. During exercise events lasting more than one hour, consume carbohydrates and/or electrolytes in a fluid replacement solution; this will not significantly impair water delivery to the body and may enhance performance.

6. Carbohydrates should be ingested at a rate of 30 to 60 grams per hour (120 to 240 calories from carbohydrates per hour) to maintain oxidation of carbohydrates and to delay fatigue during intense exercise lasting longer than one hour. The carbohydrates in the beverage can be sugars (glucose or sucrose) or starch (e.g., maltodextrin), as found in commonly available sports drinks.

7. Try sports drinks that contain sodium (0.5 to 0.7 grams per liter of water) if exercise lasts longer than one hour; they may be advantageous in enhancing palatability, improving the desire to drink, promoting fluid retention, and possibly preventing low blood volume.

# Eating and Exercise

To get the optimum benefits from your workout, consider the following factors for eating well before, during, and after exercise.

## Pre-Exercise Nutrition

In general, the pre-exercise meal should focus on the provision of carbohydrates and fluids. See the following table for a sample balanced pre-exercise meal. Consider several goals for your pre-exercise meal:

- **To obtain sufficient energy.** Make certain you obtain sufficient energy to see you through much of the exercise session that will follow the meal. Inadequate energy intake may lead to light-headedness, blurred vision, early fatigue, and loss of competitive attitude.

- **To prevent feelings of hunger.** Feeling hungry is a sign that blood sugar may be low. Low blood sugar could impair muscle function and is related to central nervous system fatigue.

- **To maintain adequate hydration.** Take in sufficient amounts of fluids to make certain you begin exercise in a fully hydrated state; this is important for performance and endurance.

- **To eat familiar foods.** Only consume foods you know make you feel good and do not cause any kind of gastrointestinal (GI) distress. If you are exercising in a country you have never been to before, you may be tempted to try unfamiliar local foods. Do not do that until after you have exercised.

- **To avoid large quantities of raw fruits and vegetables.** Raw fruits and vegetables may form gases, leading to GI distention and distress. In particular, foods in the cabbage family (such as cabbage, broccoli, cauliflower, Brussels sprouts, mustard greens, and kohlrabi) appear to pose particular problems. Eating cooked vegetables or fruit juices does not appear to lead to these kinds of problems.

- **To time your meal properly.** Time your pre-exercise meal so that you have adequate time for food to leave the stomach before the initiation of exercise. Because fats cause a delay in gastric emptying, fat in the pre-exercise meal should be kept as low as possible. Ideally, you should finish a high-carbohydrate

## Sample Pre-Exercise Meal*

| | |
|---|---|
| 2 cups spaghetti | 395 calories |
| 3/4 cup meatless spaghetti sauce | 203 calories |
| 2 tbsp parmesan cheese | 46 calories |
| 3/4 cup tossed salad | 1 calorie |
| 1 tbsp low-fat salad dressing | 67 calories |
| 2 dinner rolls | 156 calories |
| 1 cup apple juice | 116 calories |
| 2 cups water | 0 calories |
| **Totals: 69% carbohydrates; 11% protein; 20% fat; 984 calories** | |

*High in carbohydrates, moderate in protein, and low in fat

meal 3.5 to 4.0 hours before exercise if the meal is large and 2 to 3 hours before exercise if the meal is small. If fat constitutes more than 25 percent of total energy in the meal, the timing of the meal should be changed so that it is further removed from the time of exercise. Light, carbohydrate-based snacks (such as crackers) may be consumed within one hour of exercise. Sports beverages may be consumed at any time before and during exercise.

# Nutrition During Exercise

Any activity that lasts for an hour or longer places high demands on your stored energy levels. Carbohydrate consumption during activity will delay fatigue and improve performance. There is also scientific evidence suggesting that power athletes and those involved in "stop-and-go" activities can benefit from consumption of carbohydrate-containing sports beverages, even if the duration of the activity is less than one hour. The type of activity determines whether the carbohydrate should be in liquid or solid form. Several research studies have demonstrated the improved performance potential of ingesting carbohydrates during activity, so this should be an important strategy for all persons involved in regular physical activity.

Activity of moderate intensity causes a somewhat reduced (60 to 70 percent of normal) blood flow to the stomach, but the exerciser is still able to digest food in this state. Long-distance bicyclists, skiers, and ultra-marathon runners, who are working at moderate intensity over long distances, often show a preference for both solid foods (for example, bananas and bread) and sports beverages combined. Moderately intense activity involving bouncing may leave exercisers uncomfortable if solid food is consumed.

High-intensity activity dramatically reduces blood flow to the stomach (to 20 percent of normal), so solid foods are not well tolerated. Exercisers involved in these activities should plan to consume sports beverages to maintain energy and hydration. Some people do not like consuming sports beverages or foods during activity because they fear this will cause gastrointestinal (GI) problems. However, it has been demonstrated that inadequate energy and fluid intake is more likely to cause GI problems. Regular exercisers should learn to consume carbohydrate-containing sports beverages during physical activity to ensure that their hydration state is maintained and to keep a constant flow of carbohydrates entering the system.

## Post-Exercise Nutrition

Muscles are very receptive to replacing stored carbohydrate energy (glycogen) within the first one or two hours after exercise because of a high level of a circulating enzyme (glycogen synthetase) that aids this process. For those who work out on consecutive days or who have multi-day consecutive competitions, replenishing energy stores immediately after exercise is a good strategy for ensuring an optimal energy level the following day. Also, fluids must be replaced as soon after exercise as possible.

If you exercise vigorously, you should consume 200 to 400 calories from carbohydrates immediately following physical activity, and then an additional 200 to 400 calories from carbohydrates within the next several hours (see the following table). Those who have difficulty eating foods immediately following exhaustive exercise should try high-carbohydrate liquid supplements, which have the added benefit of providing needed fluids.

### Examples of High-Carbohydrate Foods That Can Be Consumed Following Exercise

| Food | Calories | % Carbohydrate |
| --- | --- | --- |
| 1 bagel | 165 | 76 |
| 2 slices bread | 135 | 81 |
| 1 cup pasta | 215 | 81 |
| 3 cups popcorn | 70 | 79 |
| 1 baked potato | 100 | 88 |
| 1 apple | 80 | 100 |
| 1 orange | 65 | 100 |
| 1 cup vegetable juice | 55 | 93 |

# Putting It All Together

Excellent health requires a balance between how much and how intensely you exercise, and the amounts and kinds of foods and fluids you consume. Nutrients work together, so too much of one may lead to difficulties with others. To ensure a "balance," it is important to consume a wide variety of foods (this strategy provides exposure to a wide spectrum of nutrients) and try to avoid a monotonous intake of the same few foods. Eating the same foods day in and day out is not only boring but it is almost guaranteed to eventually lead to malnutrition because no single food provides all the nutrients needed to stay healthy. Don't get caught up in the belief that if a small quantity of nutrient is good for you, more must be better. An excessive intake of one nutrient may be just as bad for you as an inadequate intake of another nutrient.

Again, nutrient balance is a key to good health. Finally, keeping fluid levels balanced is also critical to achieving good health. So here is your strategy: Eat frequent, nutritionally well-balanced and varied meals; drink plenty of fluids (especially water); engage in plenty of exercise; and take time to discover what energy balance works best for you!

CHAPTER

## 3

# Getting Ready
# to Exercise

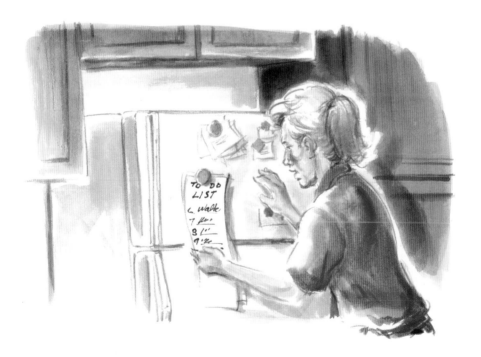

I n the first chapter, we reviewed the major physical, mental,
and emotional health benefits that you can derive from getting regular exercise. As you have seen, the physical health benefits are many. But as you begin to think seriously about adopting
this new lifestyle, you should know that for many of us who exercise regularly, it is nice to know about the physical health benefits, but the mental and emotional benefits may be what really
make us continue our regimen.

If you are reading this book, you are at least thinking about becoming a regular exerciser. In this chapter, we will share with you the major first steps you should take to help ensure the greatest chance of your success.

# Natural History of Healthy Behavior Change

If you are leading a sedentary lifestyle, engaging in no job-related or leisure-time extraneous physical exertion, then exercising regularly will obviously be a big change for you. But can a person say, at any given time in life, "OK, I'm going to start a program now; I will stick with it indefinitely; and a lifetime pattern of regular exercise will be the result," and be assured of success? For most people, the answer to that question is no.

We hope that you are ready now. We hope that is why you are reading this book. But it might not be the right time right now. Maybe the right time for you will be three months or six months or even two years from now. And that's OK. Even if you find after reading this book that you are indeed not ready to start now, you would have a leg up, or should we say you would be a step ahead, when the right time does come.

The health status of each of us changes over time. It is the very rare person who can be entirely healthy at any one time. A sound aphorism that applies to all health-promoting lifestyle or behavior changes is, "We can never be perfect; we can always get better." In the course of our own lifetimes each of us will engage in some particular aspect of "getting better," such as becoming a regular exerciser, but *when* this happens varies widely from person to person. We will repeat this because it is an important lesson: *Perfection is not the objective here.* Different people change at different rates of speed at different times in their lives. We hope, and likely you do as well, that you are ready to start exercising regularly and stay with it now. But if you are like just about everybody else, if you are not ready right now you may very well be able to do it down the road, when you are ready.

# First Steps

We all have to begin somewhere. However, no exercise program will work for you if you just jump right in with no plan, no goals, and no idea of where you are and how far you need or want to go. The first steps to take before you start the physical part of your fitness program are mental ones: *assessment, goal setting,* and *motivation.*

## Assessment

You may be surprised to learn that the first steps in getting started properly do not have to do with such matters as what sport, what equipment, and what workout schedule you should follow. Those are all important, but the most important steps to take at the beginning are a series of mental ones. You need to do some serious thinking if your chances of success in becoming a regular exerciser are to be as high as they can be.

There are no scientific studies on what we are about to say (and indeed such studies would be difficult and expensive to do), but observation tells us that most people who achieve long-term success do not plunge right in at the beginning on one particular exercise program, sport, or schedule (such as those described in chapters 5 and 6) without exercising their minds first. The first mental task to do is self-assessment. In the next chapter, we take you through the ACSM Fitness Assessment, which relates to physical fitness. But before you complete that assessment, there is the matter of mental fitness and readiness.

Where are you now in your physical activity level? Have you tried regular exercise before and failed to stick with it? What do you estimate your potential to be to stick with an exercise program? (Realism is very important here.) What unmet personal needs are you thinking about attempting to meet? Are you ready, really ready, to try it? We will get into these types of questions in some detail in the following discussion.

## Long-Term Goal Setting

The second mental step is for you to set long-term goals. For example, what would you like to accomplish? To look better? Feel better? Feel better about yourself? Reduce your future risk of contracting one or more of the diseases associated with a sedentary lifestyle? Lose weight? Become fit for fitness' own sake? Then, why do you want to accomplish what you want to accomplish? Going back to self-assessment, what current unmet personal needs are you hoping to meet? Very important, for whom will you make the effort—yourself or someone else?

If you try to become a regular exerciser in response to an external influence, such as a family member or a job situation, then anger, guilt, frustration, injury, and quitting are much more likely to be the outcome of your efforts than the happy, healthy, gradual, and comfortable incorporation of regular exercise into your life.

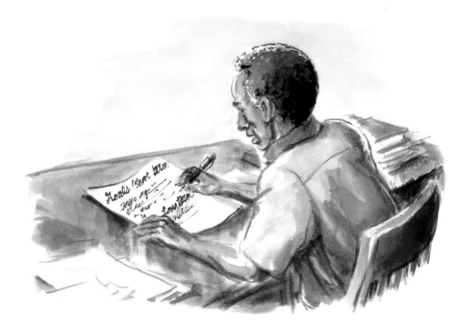

# Motivation

The third primary mental step you need to take to give yourself the best chance of achieving success is mobilizing your motivation. As we will see, motivation is a process, not a thing. Thus, no one person can give it to another. Neither can it be found packaged in a pill or a machine. If one is not motivated, it does not mean that they haven't got the "stuff." It simply means that the motivational process for the given desired change hasn't been mobilized. It is through the process of mobilizing motivation that people make changes for themselves. Dealing with negative thoughts should begin that process.

Often, the first thoughts popping into the head of anyone even thinking about the possibility of exercising on a regular basis are along the lines of "It's too hard. I'm not an athlete and never will be. It's not worth the effort. It'll kill my knees. It won't be fun. I'll hate it." You should know that such first thoughts do not need to be your last on the subject of regular exercise. Many people have started from the same place and have actually come not only to tolerate but also to truly enjoy the activity. This is especially so if they have taken the time to go through the three primary mental exercises we have just introduced.

# Permanent Time Requirements of Regular Exercise

It is an unavoidable fact of life that becoming a regular exerciser by definition requires that you spend time on it, regularly, for the rest of your life. Whatever amount of time you are able to devote to it, right now you are spending it doing something else. Furthermore, very few of the other lifestyle or behavior changes you could make to improve your health share that characteristic. If you stop smoking, change the way you eat, manage your weight better, always wear your automobile seatbelt, or exercise regularly, it is only the last lifestyle change that requires a significant amount of extra time.

To be a regular exerciser you must find time in your life schedule on an ongoing basis. It may be only two or three hours a week for the exercise time, plus another hour or so each time for changing clothes, showering, and getting to the pool or gym. But those are three to six hours per week that you are now spending on something else. We will come back to this subject in a bit more detail later in this chapter. And finally, we will take a look at how to go about judging your rate and degree of success in this new endeavor.

# Your Self-Assessment Plan

Now that we have had an overview of what is in this chapter, let us turn our attention in some detail to the first mental task you need to undertake to begin properly on the road to becoming a regular exerciser: self-assessment of where you are in your life, in terms of exercising, now. The mental tasks are connected with one another and with the ongoing process of behavior change in a continuous, self-reinforcing, feedback loop. Self-assessment, as we shall see, is closely connected to goal setting. The elements of self-assessment at this level are of your mind, the condition of your body as you see it, and of your previous experience. You want to ask yourself several questions:

- What is it about my body and mind that I am unhappy with that could be positively affected by exercising regularly?
- What is it that I might or do want to change? And why?
- Would I really like to change, even if it means giving up something I am accustomed to?
- Do I think that I can mobilize the mental strength (and it does take mental strength —there are no magic bullets to significantly change a personal health-related behavior), if that is what I want or need to do?
- What is it that I like about my body? Don't like? Would like to change?
- What is my body self-image, truly? Does it at all correspond to reality as others tell me that reality is?
- Am I being realistic about this?

- What has my previous experience with personal health behavior change been? Good? Bad? Some success? None? Will that help me this time around? What can I learn from experience that will help this time?

As you ask yourself these questions, think intrinsically: What is your image of yourself? How do you think of yourself—good-looking? Attractive? Not attractive? Healthy? Unhealthy? What do you see when you look in the mirror? What kinds of feelings do those images elicit? And when you see, for instance, "fat," do others say that that is a true reflection of reality? If you are planning to exercise to help in weight loss or simply to shape up a currently out-of-shape body, will you be able to use the facts that smaller clothing now fits and that your waist is getting smaller (that's at least smaller, if not small) as measures of success, rather than scale weight (which might or might not change much, even as you are redistributing body mass)?

How much weight would you have to lose to get below the upper limit of the normal weight range for your age, height, and sex? Would that make you truly happier or might you feel the urge to lose even more weight? If you are going to exercise primarily for weight loss, is your true goal to become really thin rather than somewhat thinner? Are you in reality looking for the

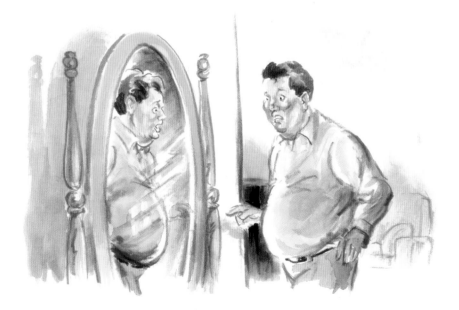

"perfect body," something few of us could achieve, even if there were such a thing? And if so, why? Answering these questions will be important in defining your long-term goals and mobilizing your motivation.

## Am I *Really* Ready to Begin?

Most people will use both objective (something you can measure) and subjective (something you feel) criteria in coming to the decision to begin a program of behavior change. Taking an overweight person as the example, the objective criterion might be the measure of overall body size called the *body mass index* (*BMI*) (page 79). This is a number derived from a formula that factors in both weight and height to represent a person's degree of "fatness." An overweight person could, for example, find her BMI number on the BMI table; if the number were above normal she could then decide to attempt to lose weight and body fat. On the other hand, subjective criteria such as dissatisfaction with being out of breath after climbing a flight of stairs, or, for cigarette smokers the internalization of the increased relative risk of developing lung cancer, can also lead you to become a regular exerciser or to quit using cigarettes.

The reality is that few overweight people would come to the conclusion that they are too heavy using objective criteria like their BMI alone, and thus decide to do something about their weight, really do something about it this time. That is, not too many people wake up one day, go to the BMI table, determine that their BMI is 10 units too high, and then say, "OK, the time has come to lose some weight. Tomorrow I'm going to start a comprehensive program of regular exercise and healthy eating." Much more likely is a scenario in which after quite some time of being overweight one finally feels, deep down inside, that the time has come to lose weight. Then, perhaps after several previous failures, she is prepared to seriously attempt to do so, over an extended time. For example, such a person might say to herself, "I'm just tired of being overweight and out of shape. I know how and why I got this way, and I have decided to take control of my body and my life. I'm finally going to do something about my weight and shape that will work in the long run. I know what the sacrifices are. I know how tough it's going to be, but I also have finally convinced myself that it is worth making them. Yes, it's going to be tough, but I'm going to do it."

Another of the several keys to success is not starting until you have reached that point in your mind's journey when you are truly ready to start. You need to make sure that you have done your mental assessment carefully and accurately. You must be and feel ready to go.

## Setting Goals

In this book, we use two versions of the term *goal*. *Long-term goal,* a term you will encounter frequently in this chapter, refers to a medium- to long-range desired outcome of a lifestyle or behavior change activity, such as becoming a regular exerciser. A long-term goal is a reason that you have provided to yourself for doing it. Some examples are as follows: "I would like to feel better and also feel better about myself"; "I would like to look better"; "I would like to get into shape for once in my life"; "I would eventually like to be able to run a 10K road race."

The term *short-term goal* refers to specific outcomes of a specific set of exercises or a workout schedule: "By the end of next week, I'm going to able to walk nonstop at a 15-minute-per-mile pace for 30 minutes"; "Over the next four weeks, I'm going to work up to doing five workouts per week from the schedule that I have worked out for myself from the information in chapter 6"; "Over the next three months, my aim is to double the weight I can lift now in a bench press."

The most important element in undertaking any personal behavior change is long-term goal setting. The process of long-term goal setting enables you to focus, indeed forces you to focus, on the task at hand, to mobilize your motivation around self-established, expected outcomes that are realistic and meaningful to you. By asking yourself these questions, you will lay the foundation for planning and organizing a specific exercise program (choosing from the options laid out for you in chapters 5 and 6) that is relevant to you and has meaning for you.

As we noted in the introduction to this chapter, long-term goal setting thus encompasses knowing what you want to do, why you want to do it, for whom you are doing it, and what you expect to get out of it. Setting goals and taking some time to do so requires you to focus on the reasons you want to change, not just the change process itself. Setting goals establishes the link between thought and action that characterizes the motivational process.

In setting your long-term goals, you will address questions such as the following:

- What is it that I want to do in regular exercise?
- Why do I want to do it?
- Why do I want to do this now?
- For whom do I want to make the change(s)—myself or someone else?
- Do I want to feel better? Look better? Feel better about myself? Reduce my future risk of disease? Become healthier? Get into competitive sports at some level?
- Am I being realistic about what I would like to accomplish?

A very important reason for carefully setting your long-term goals is that doing so will make it much easier to stick with the program when those quitting thoughts arise (and they almost invariably do). Because then it will not be simply, "I've got to stick with this because I've got to stick with this," but rather, "I've got to stick with this for the reasons I started doing what I'm doing in the first place, and deep down I know that I very much still want to get to where I originally decided I want to be."

Be realistic in setting your long-term as well as your short-term goals. The initial goals you set must be reasonable ones for you at the time you set them. Recognize that what you consider to be realistic is likely to change over time, as exercising becomes a regular part of your life. But nothing can kill a change process faster than the setting of unrealistic, unachievable long-term goals.

If at the outset you set goals that are truly beyond your abilities by any stretch of the imagination (e.g., "After starting from scratch as a runner, within three months I will finish a marathon"), doing so will almost invariably lead to frustration, pain, injury, and quitting. Setting your goals too low (e.g., "For as long as I exercise regularly, I will only walk, only at my regular walking pace, and for not more than 20 minutes at a time"), on the other hand, will almost invariably lead to boredom. Both boredom and the placing of too-low physical demands on the body are major factors in the failure to achieve any of the desired physical and mental outcomes of regular exercise.

In setting goals for exercise, we must recognize the role our genes play in determining what we can do. A strong genetic component is involved in the determination of body shape and size, potential strength, ability to increase muscle bulk by weightlifting, and achieving speed in any sport. At the same time, we must emphasize that within our genetic limitations we can make significant changes in physical fitness, strength, speed to some extent, and certainly sports and athletic skills. Thus your goals can be, and in many cases should be, changed over time, but gradually and realistically.

## Exploring Limits and Recognizing Limitations

Thus we arrive at another favorite aphorism: "Explore your limits; recognize your limitations." Once you have embarked on your journey to becoming a regular exerciser, you may find yourself taken to places in mind and body you never previously dreamed possible for you. A couch potato may, eventually, become a marathoner if he wants to be one. A "97-pound weakling" may eventually develop a nicely formed body outline with a significant increase in strength. An uncoordinated large-bodied person may eventually become a group exercise leader or cycling instructor, regardless of final weight. Getting to such previously unimagined or unimaginable heights involves exploring your limits in physical activity. Many who have tried such exploration have in the end been very pleasantly surprised with the outcome.

At the same time you are exploring your limits, you should take care to recognize and accept your physical limitations. Speed, strength, muscular bulk, flexibility, and gracefulness are in part achieved through training and practice. But as noted, they are in significant part achieved as a result of genetic makeup.

Exactly what proportion of each achievement is determined by your personal gene pool and what proportion by your effort is of course not as yet known. But few of us have the genetic makeup to enable us to be either a world-class athlete or a world-class model, no matter how much work we do. Thus, not setting goals of that sort, even in relative terms, will be liberating and empowering. Realism in goal setting will go a long way toward enhancing the chances of success in behavior-change efforts. As long as you recognize your limitations (for example, in terms of speed), exploration of what your true limits are (for example, in terms of distance) may lead you into a territory of athletic achievement that you had never before contemplated.

## Getting Motivated

Most people have a general idea of what they mean when they say, "I've got to get motivated," or "My motivation is high." But few of us can immediately put into words exactly what we mean when we use the term *motivation*. Indeed, even among professionals, many who use it frequently do not bother to define it. This could be because it is assumed that everyone just knows how it is defined, even if that is often not the case. But because motivation is such an important element in achieving success in behavior change, being familiar with a written definition is helpful. One definition is "Motivation is a mental process that links an emotion, feeling, desire, idea, or intellectual understanding, or a recognized psychological, physiological, or health need, to the taking of one or more actions."

In the short form, "Motivation is a mental process that links a thought or a feeling to an action." When we talk either about being motivated or lacking motivation to engage in a behavior change such as becoming a regular exerciser, we are referring to the process of our mind that will impel us to undertake that action. Thus, motivation is always related to action. The key, then, is not the acquisition of motivation from somebody or somewhere else. It is, rather, the mobilization of the motivational process that exists in virtually all of us. Motivation mobilization is the third essential element of the pathway to success in any lifestyle or behavior-change effort.

Put another way, motivation is intangible. It is not a thing that can or must be acquired somewhere or from someone else. It is, to repeat, a mental process. Striving to be healthy is essential both for self- and for species preservation. Thus getting motivated is not a matter of developing or importing a mind-state. It is, rather, a matter of activating a process of the mind that is present but presently inoperative: of locating it, of mobilizing it, and of removing the barriers to its activation.

## External Versus Internal Motivation

The scientific literature is clear that in most cases, if it is to be effective, motivation must be internally directed. Thus, if the motivational process is to be effectively activated, there should be thoughts along the lines of, "I want to do this for me—to look better, feel better, get healthier, feel better about myself—not for anyone else."

Externally originated motivation, "I'm doing this for my [spouse, boyfriend or girlfriend, children or parents, employer or coworkers]" almost invariably leads to one or more of the following: guilt feelings, anxiety, anger, and frustration. Often the next step after that is quitting. The one exception to the inner-directed rule is when you can honestly say, "I'm doing this for someone else because it will make me feel good and feel good about myself to make them happy." But even in this case the primary motivation mobilizer is still internal.

If you want to look better, feel better, feel better about yourself, and get healthier for yourself, for no one else, then you have inner motivation. If you view approval by others for making the behavior change and achieving its desired outcome(s) simply as an extra benefit of doing so, then too, you have inner motivation. With inner motivation you will be able to take control of your physical activity pattern and level, mode of eating, use of drugs such as nicotine and alcohol, approach to managing stress, and so on and so forth, and hence achieve health-promoting and disease-preventing changes in your body, yourself, and the way you live your life.

## Guilt as a Motivation Mobilizer

When contemplating a positive lifestyle or behavior change, some people have such thoughts as *I have to, I ought to,* and *I should* (in contrast with *I want to, I would like to, it would make me feel good to*). *Have to, ought to,* and *should* are all representations of a potential feeling of guilt, which is a painful feeling of self-reproach resulting from a belief that you have done something wrong or immoral.

Much experience has shown that this guilt-inducing "you-gotta" approach, whether self- or other-inflicted, if it elicits guilt feelings, has been generally found to be counterproductive. Guilt feelings often elicit (in psychological terms) resistance or denial. In lay language, those terms translate as, "I don't want to," and, "Problem? What problem?"

Furthermore, feeling guilty about anything without a fairly quick resolution of those feelings often leads to frustration and then anger. Most of us do not like feeling either angry or frustrated on an ongoing basis. If feeling guilty is the reason we started doing something new in the first place, then the presence of those thoughts is likely to lead us to quit doing what we're doing, because doing so will be the easiest way to get rid of the anger and frustration.

### Five Keys to Mobilizing Motivation

1. Understand motivation.
2. Undertake self-assessment.
3. Set long-term goals that are realistically achievable.
4. Be willing to explore your limits while recognizing your limitations.
5. Put these steps together to take control of your life.

Taking control of your life is absolutely critical to locating, unblocking, and mobilizing your motivation. Having gone through steps 1 through 3, you say to yourself, "Yes, I can do this; I want to do this; and I know why. I can run my eating pattern instead of having it run me. I can take control of my time so that I can engage in a reasonable amount of regular exercise. I can do so because I truly have worked out the whys and wherefores for myself."

For many people, the mental act of taking control is itself a central element both in beginning a behavior change effort and in sticking with it. You have many choices to make: whether to undertake a change process at all, what long-term goals to set, how precisely to do it, and what sort of exercise program to begin with (we, of course, recommend the one discussed in chapters 5 and 6 of this book). Taking control is empowering, as is the realization that you are taking control when perhaps you have not done that too often, if ever, in the past. Being able to say, "Yes, I am doing this; yes, I can do this," whatever the "this" is, can bring joy to your heart and open up new horizons for you.

It is important to reemphasize that motivation is almost always there in most of us, whether or not it is currently mobilized. But we do have to unleash it within ourselves. No one else can do that for us. Only when the connection is made between the thought or feeling and the action is motivation mobilized.

Among the common blocks to the motivation process that accompany so many attempts at behavior change are the thoughts, "I really don't want to do this, I know I'll just never be able to get started, I just know I don't have the time." There is no magic answer for getting through these blocks, but using the "Five Keys" can certainly help.

## Ambivalence

Ambivalence can be a major factor inhibiting your ability to mobilize your motivation. Ambivalence is a state of mind characterized by coexisting but conflicting feelings about a contemplated action, another person, or a situation in which you find yourself. This state of mind often leads to formulations such as the following:

- I want to/I don't want to.
- I know I can do this/I really don't think I can do this.
- One day I want to/the next day I don't.

Feeling ambivalent from time to time is a perfectly healthy state of mind. Virtually everyone who even thinks about making a major (and sometimes even a minor) change in his or her life experiences it. But to get on with the change process you have to deal with ambivalence. The inner conflict has to be resolved. Allowing it to paralyze decision making is a problem. What you do in response to the feelings determines their impact. Handled in the right way, the process of resolving ambivalent feelings itself can actually help you to get started down the road to success in changing a health-related behavior. The first key to effectively dealing with ambivalence is to simply accept that it will always be present to some extent. Sometimes the ambivalent feelings will be weaker and sometimes stronger.

To get started with a lifestyle or behavior change such as becoming a regular exerciser, you will have to be able to get at least partly on the track that already exists in your mind that leads to thoughts like, *"Yes, I would like to change; yes I can change."* Ambivalence does not have to be completely resolved to get started, however. Even someone who already is a regular exerciser may occasionally encounter negative feelings ranging from just not wanting to get out of bed in time to work out on a particular morning to thinking, *"Why am I doing this, anyway?"* But then they deal with the particular reluctance (by either overcoming it or, on occasion, giving in to it), or the general doubt (by reviewing their self-assessment and goal-setting processes), and they continue on, anyway.

Those thoughts are OK—as long as you do not get so far away from the program that what has already been accomplished is undone. If ambivalence destroys commitment, then that is a problem. However, if it simply questions commitment, if it does nothing more than lead to a temporary detour now and again, it can even be a good thing, leading you to strengthen your resolve to proceed forward. Again, as in motivation mobilization, self-assessment and goal setting are powerful tools for dealing with ambivalence.

## Willpower

Given that willpower in terms of personal health-related behavior means the conscious mental ability to follow through on plans to change it, or to maintain a change once it is made, then willpower is absolutely essential to success. Do not let anyone or any book (such as those "no-willpower exercise plans") tell you anything different. In the context of your personal health, using willpower simply means mobilizing your mental capacity to make a change in the carrying out of a physical act—nothing more and nothing less. And that is precisely what the person changing his personal behavior needs to do to make the desired change(s). It's that simple and that complicated.

## Making the Time

As we have noted at the beginning of this chapter, becoming a regular exerciser intrudes on your time for the rest of your life. You should not sweep this aspect of the enterprise under the rug. You need to examine it carefully.

How are you spending your time now? Can you give up four hours of television a week? Can you get up 45 minutes earlier four days a week (including the two weekend days) and cut down on dawdling time by 15 minutes on each of those days? Can your spouse, for example, do some of the food shopping and cooking and help with some household chores? If necessary, can you find some time during your workday to squeeze in time for working out? Better yet, can you take advantage of a health promotion program that many employers now sponsor, or can you make a suggestion to start one if it is not currently offered at your workplace?

The details of the ACSM Fitness Program for getting on and staying with a modestly demanding program of regular exercise that is right for you are to be found in chapter 6. But those "There's nothing to it; you can easily find the time" or "It really doesn't take any time at all" messages that accompany some exercise program recommendations, like those "no willpower" messages that accompany many weight-loss programs, are not to be believed. Regular exercise to a level that will provide significant benefits both for feeling good now and for future risk-factor reduction does take time. Most people can find the time. But you have to have a plan; you have to want to do it; and you have to be able to take control and mobilize your motivation—for few people it is that easy, at least in the beginning. But the advice and suggestions we provide in this book will make it easier.

# Measuring Success

And finally, under the subject of getting ready to exercise, to which this chapter is devoted, it is a good idea to spend a bit of time at the beginning thinking about how you are going to define *success* for yourself. First, you should make sure that the definition of success you use for yourself is entirely interlinked with the long-term goals you have set for yourself. Furthermore, as we have said more than once, you need to make sure that those goals are realistic at the time you set them, in terms of your realistically available time, your present physical status, and your present mind-set. Once goals are realistically delineated, then what constitutes success can be realistically delineated as well.

First, remember that what constitutes success varies from person to person. Second (and this is part of the concept of the natural history of healthy behavior change that we talked about at the beginning of this chapter), within each person what constitutes success can vary over time, too. Third, recall the saying, "Explore your limits; recognize your limitations." This has particular applicability to the concept that success is relative. Exploring your limits, gradually and realistically, especially in the area of regular exercise, can lead you to achievements not even remotely contemplated previously.

C H A P T E R

# 4

# Assessing Your Fitness: The ACSM Fitness Test

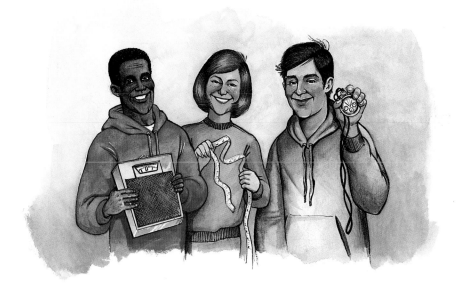

**H**ealth-related physical fitness includes aerobic fitness, muscular fitness, flexibility, and body composition. Each of these important concepts was introduced in chapter 1. For us to determine a good starting point for your lifelong program of good health and regular exercise, it is important to do some tests of your current health status. We should caution you, however: If you have experienced any medical situation requiring a physician's care, or if you have been told to reduce your physical activity for any reason, you should consult your doctor before beginning an exercise program. Most of us do not fit into this category. However, it is always a good idea to start with a complete medical examination by a physician before beginning an exercise program.

Now it is time to discover more about your own personal fitness so you can establish both short-term and long-term goals. The ACSM Fitness Test is a series of four assessments that you can use to evaluate your current level of physical fitness. The tests are easy to perform and can be completed in less than one hour. As you take the test, you will record your results for each assessment on the sheets provided at the end of this chapter. We have also included the results for "Frank" and for "Jackie," two models who have agreed to include their data. Your results will let you know at which level of the ACSM Fitness Program you should begin exercising.

# Why Fitness Testing Is a Good Idea

You discovered in chapter 1 that regular exercise produces a variety of important physical changes. But, changes are often difficult to recognize because most occur gradually. To identify your rate of progress, take the ACSM Fitness Test at regular intervals throughout the year. It will also allow you to understand the effort required for you to see positive results from your exercise program. As your scores in the ACSM Fitness Test improve, you will enjoy a greater feeling of accomplishment and satisfaction. Plan to take the ACSM Fitness Test after about six weeks of your initial program, then at about three-to-six-month intervals. Plan to repeat the test again on the one-year anniversary of your first day of the program, and see the wonderful changes that have happened to you.

# Are You Ready to Begin?

The activities in the ACSM Fitness Book are designed for adults of all ages who want to begin an exercise program. For most people, physical activity of moderate intensity is not dangerous, and no medical evaluation is necessary. However, certain individuals should consult with a physician before they begin exercising and before completing the assessments in this chapter. Take a few minutes to answer the questions in the pre-participation checklist. If you answer "yes" to any of these items, we advise you to seek a medical opinion about the type of exercise that is safe and appropriate for you before you start with this program.

## Pre-Participation Checklist

| | Yes | No |
|---|---|---|
| 1. Has your doctor ever said you have a heart condition <u>and</u> that you should only do physical activity recommended by a doctor? | | |
| 2. Do you feel pain in your chest when you do physical activity? | | |
| 3. In the past month, have you had chest pain when you were not doing physical activity? | | |
| 4. Do you lose your balance because of dizziness or do you ever lose consciousness? | | |
| 5. Do you have a bone or joint problem (for example, back, knee, or hip) that could be made worse by a change in your physical activity? | | |
| 6. Is your doctor currently prescribing drugs (for example, water pills) for your blood pressure or heart condition? | | |
| 7. Do you know of <u>any other reason</u> why you should not do physical activity? | | |

Excerpted from the 2002 revised version of the Physical Activity Readiness Questionnaire (PAR-Q). Reprinted with permission of the Canadian Society for Exercise Physiology.

# Gathering Your Supplies

The four assessments that make up the ACSM Fitness Test are the Rockport One-Mile (1.6 km) Walking Test for aerobic fitness, a push-up test for muscular fitness, a sit-and-reach test for flexibility, and determination of your body composition through the body mass index (BMI) and the waist-to-hip ratio. You can complete three of the four items in the ACSM Fitness Test in your own home. The walking test requires a flat, measured walking surface, which you should be able to find at a neighborhood school or college track, a community fitness center, a community park, or a sidewalk along a flat street (you will have to measure the distance by driving your car along the street and note the distance with appropriate landmarks). You will also need to gather some basic equipment to complete the tests. This would include a watch with a second hand, or a stopwatch; a tape measure; a scale, to measure your weight; a yardstick; and adhesive tape (any type will do).

You can do these tests on your own, but it is best to take the test with a friend or relative. You can help each other do the assessments, and your measurements may be more accurate. Taking the tests together is also a great way to involve your friend or relative in the exercise program, and exercising with someone else is an excellent way to ensure that both of you stick with your program.

To take the ACSM Fitness Test, it is best to wear appropriate clothes and athletic shoes, but any comfortable shoes are fine. We recommend a warm-up suit or elastic-waist slacks or shorts and a T-shirt, but you can wear any loose-fitting clothing.

After you have dressed appropriately, gathered all the equipment, and found your measured walking site, you can begin the assessments. As with any exercise, the ACSM Fitness Test begins with an appropriate warm-up. The warm-up is important because it allows your heart rate and respiration to increase gradually and your muscles to loosen, and it warms your body, all of which should make your assessments and exercise easier. An appropriate warm up includes light aerobic activity, such as slow walking and slow stretching exercises; see those presented in the level 1 flexibility program beginning on page 109.

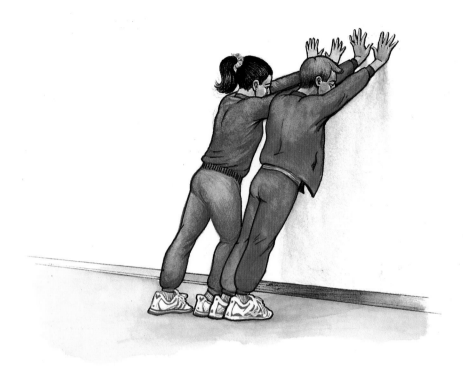

# Ready, Set, Go!

Now, let's see if you have completed all of the requirements prior to beginning this lifelong commitment to good health. Have you

- written down your personal exercise goals?
- completed the pre-participation checklist?
- answered "no" to all the questions on the pre-participation checklist, or consulted with your doctor?

If so, then you are **READY** to start! Have you

- found a friend or relative to take the test with you?
- gathered all of the testing equipment?
- warmed up appropriately?

If so, then you are **SET** to begin!
Now, **GO!** Begin your ACSM Fitness Test!

# Creating Your Personal Fitness Profile

Just as there are four components of health-related physical fitness (aerobic fitness, muscular fitness, flexibility, and body composition), there are four assessments in the ACSM Fitness Test. Assess your fitness in each of the four components. Your fitness may be high in one category but low in another category. Determining your fitness in each of the four areas will allow you to choose the appropriate exercises for your current status in each area.

As you complete each phase of the ACSM Fitness Test, record your results on your personal fitness profile. Use only the first blank space for each component when you complete the assessment for the first time. As you continue throughout the program and are ready for a retest, record your new results in the other blank spaces. When you are done with the fitness test, the profile will be finished, and you will be ready to develop a fitness program based on your results.

To illustrate exactly how the ACSM Fitness Test works and how you find your results and record your scores, Jackie (a 48-year-old female) and Frank (a 37-year-old male) will be used as models. Jackie and Frank are friends who work together. Recently, a

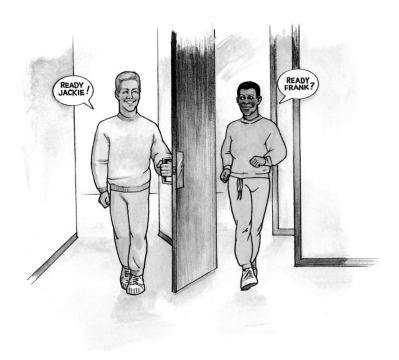

# ACSM Personal Fitness Profile
## for

_____

Your Name

| Fitness Component | Test | Date | Scores | Fitness Level and Color |
|---|---|---|---|---|
| Aerobic Fitness | Rockport 1-Mile (1.6 km) Walk | | Time: HR: | |
| | | | Time: HR: | |
| | | | Time: HR: | |
| | | | Time: HR: | |
| Muscular Fitness | Push-Ups | | Number: | |
| | | | Number: | |
| | | | Number: | |
| | | | Number: | |
| Flexibility | Sit and Reach | | Inches: | |
| | | | Inches: | |
| | | | Inches: | |
| | | | Inches: | |
| Body Composition | Body Mass Index and Waist-to-Hip Ratio | | BMI: W/H: | |
| | | | BMI: W/H: | |
| | | | BMI: W/H: | |
| | | | BMI: W/H: | |

colleague from their office had a heart attack. Realizing it could just as easily have happened to them, Jackie and Frank decided to help each other begin and maintain a regular exercise program. They chose the ACSM Fitness Program. Both have followed our instructions so far, and now they are ready to begin the first test.

## Rockport One-Mile (1.6 km) Walking Test

### Equipment
- Flat, one-mile (1.6 km) walking surface
- Watch or stopwatch

### Preparation
- Wear comfortable, loose-fitting clothes and sturdy walking shoes.
- Avoid smoking, eating, and ingesting caffeine for at least two hours before the test. Drinking noncaffeinated beverages is encouraged.
- Practice taking your pulse. The walking test requires that you count your heart rate accurately. Practice feeling your pulse and counting your heart rate. Your pulse is located at the base of your thumb at your wrist, or at your neck, just to the side of your windpipe. Use your index and middle fingers to find your pulse, and count the number of beats for 15 seconds. Count the first beat you feel as zero (then 1, 2, 3, and so on). Multiply the number of beats you feel in 15 seconds by 4 to arrive at your heart rate per minute. It is important to measure your heart rate accurately. Have your friend or relative take your pulse at the same time and compare results. They should be the same. Practice on each other until you are sure your pulse rate is accurate.

### Procedures
1. Warm up by walking slowly for a few minutes then stretching gently using the quadriceps stretch and wall lean (page 122).
2. Look at your watch to note the time, or start the stopwatch.
3. Begin walking. Complete the distance by walking as quickly as you can.

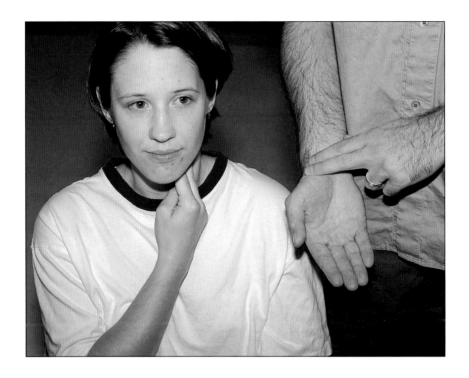

4. Immediately note the time it took to complete the distance.

5. Find your pulse and count the number of beats in 15 seconds, following the procedures outlined previously. Remember to count the first beat you feel as zero.

6. Multiply your 15-second heart rate by 4 to arrive at your heart rate per minute.

7. Record your time and heart rate on your personal fitness profile.

## *Determining Your Fitness Level*

Use the charts on pages 74 to 77 to determine your current aerobic fitness level.

- Select the chart appropriate to your sex and age.
- Find your heart rate along the left side of the chart, and draw a horizontal line across the graph at this heart rate.
- Find the time it took you to complete the distance along the bottom of the chart, and draw a straight line up the graph from that time.

- Read your aerobic fitness level at the intersection of the two lines you have just drawn.
- Once you have determined your aerobic fitness level, record it on your personal fitness profile.

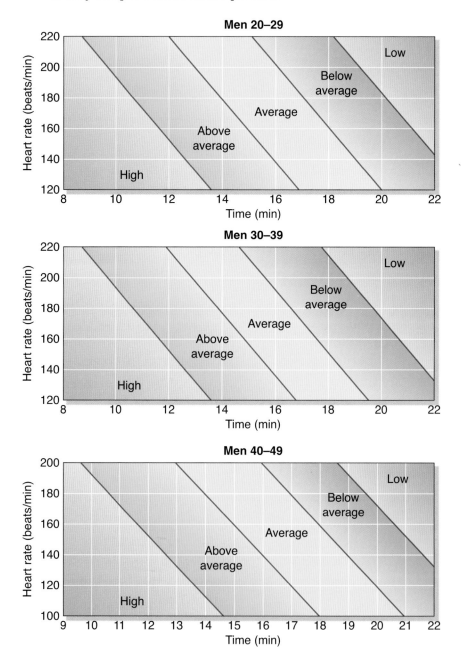

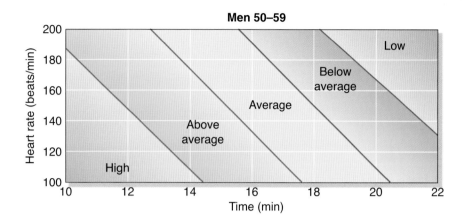

**Men 50–59**

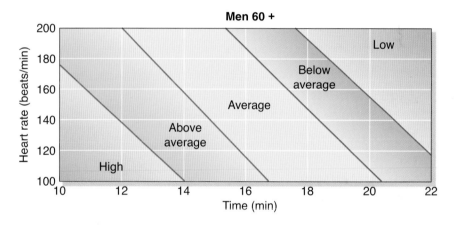

**Men 60 +**

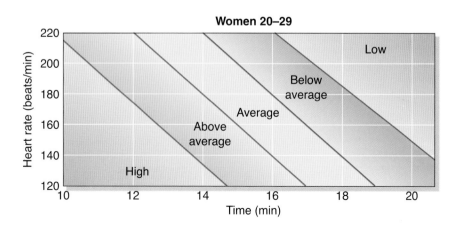

**Women 20–29**

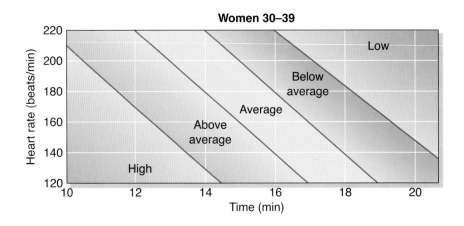

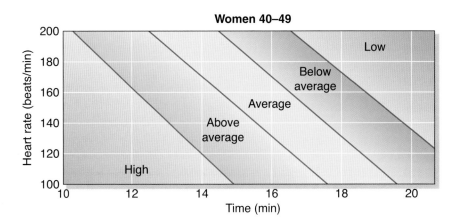

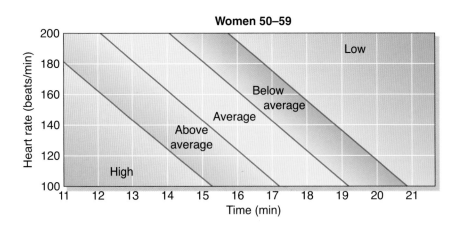

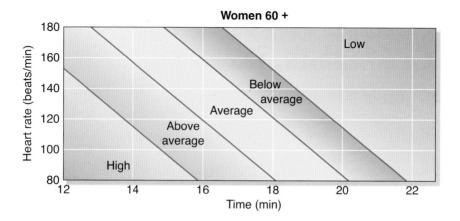

As Frank warmed up by walking and stretching on the football field encircled by their local high school track, Jackie checked that her stopwatch was working. When Frank finished his warm-up and took his place on the track, Jackie yelled, "Start!" and began her stopwatch. As Frank began walking quickly, Jackie shouted encouragement. When Frank completed his final lap around the track, Jackie stopped the watch and noted that it had taken Frank 17 minutes and 25 seconds to complete the walk. As Frank quickly found his pulse, Jackie reset the stopwatch. Again Jackie said, "Start," and Frank began to count. At the end of 15 seconds, Jackie asked Frank for his heart rate. Frank had counted 30 beats in 15 seconds (after starting with zero, then 1, 2, 3, and so on). Jackie multiplied the 15-second count by 4 to determine that Frank's heart rate was 120 beats per minute. Before they left for the track, Frank and Jackie had made copies of the personal fitness profile. Frank recorded the date, the time it took him to walk the distance, and his heart rate. After Frank had completed his walk and recorded his information, Jackie took her turn walking as Frank operated the stopwatch. Jackie finished walking in 18 minutes and 15 seconds. Her post-walk heart rate was 132 beats per minute.

Frank found the fitness chart for 30- to 39-year-old men. Because his walk took 17 minutes and 25 seconds, along the bottom of the chart he found the spot between 16 and 18 minutes. And, because his timed heart rate was 120 beats per minute, along the side of the chart he found where 120 beats would fall. He marked the first spot and drew a line across from the second spot, and he found that they intersected in the yellow area labeled "Average." Jackie found her chart for 40- to 49-year-old women. Her lines intersected in the green area labeled "Below average." Frank and Jackie recorded their fitness levels and colors on their personal fitness profiles.

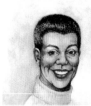

## Jackie's Results:
## 18:15, 132 bmp

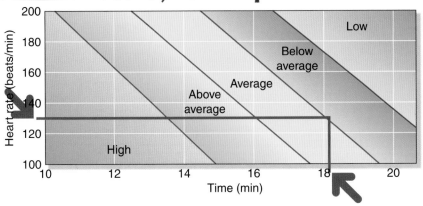

Heart rate (beats/min)

200
180
160
140
120
100

Low

Below
average

Average

Above
average

High

10   12   14   16   18   20

Time (min)

| Aerobic Fitness | Rockport 1-Mile (1.6 km) Walk | 8/5 | Time: *18:15* HR: *132 bpm* | *Below avg: Green* |
|---|---|---|---|---|
| | | | Time: HR: | |
| | | | Time: HR: | |

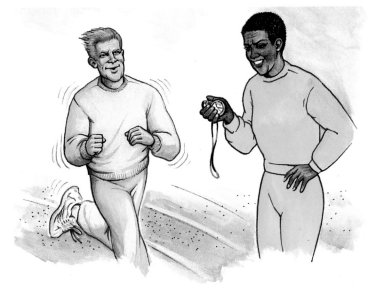

## Push-Up Test

### Equipment

- None

### Preparation

- Find a large space on the floor, clear of obstructions.
- Warm up, being sure to use the triceps stretch (page 118) and shoulder stretch (page 111).

### Procedures

- **Men:** Position yourself on the floor so that your body is straight, with your weight supported on your toes and hands. Your arms should be straight, with your hands flat on the floor, shoulder-width apart.
- **Women:** Position yourself on the floor so that your body is straight with your weight supported on your knees and hands. Your arms should be straight with your hands flat on the floor, shoulder-width apart.

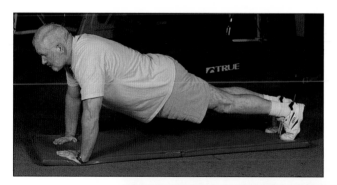

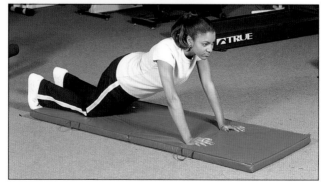

1. Lower your body until your chin touches the floor. Be sure to keep your back straight throughout the push-up. The belly should not touch the floor.
2. Push your body upward to return to the starting position.
3. Do a complete push-up each time you fully lower then raise your body to the starting position. Count the number of push-ups you are able to complete without pausing for a rest.
4. Record your score on your fitness profile.

## Determining Your Fitness Level

- Compare your score to the standards in the muscular fitness norms table. Be sure to use the standards for your age and sex.
- Once you have determined your muscular fitness level, record it on your personal fitness profile.

### Male Norms for the Push-Up Test (Number Completed)

| Rating | Age (years) | | | | |
|---|---|---|---|---|---|
| | 20–29 | 30–39 | 40–49 | 50–59 | 60–69 |
| Above average | ≥ 30 | ≥ 24 | ≥ 19 | ≥ 14 | ≥ 11 |
| Average | 24–29 | 19–23 | 13–18 | 10–13 | 9–10 |
| Below average | 18–23 | 14–18 | 10–12 | 7–9 | 6–7 |
| Low | ≤ 17 | ≤ 13 | ≤ 9 | ≤ 6 | ≤ 5 |

### Female Norms for the Push-Up Test (Number Completed)

| Rating | Age (years) | | | | |
|---|---|---|---|---|---|
| | 20–29 | 30–39 | 40–49 | 50–59 | 60–69 |
| Above average | ≥ 22 | ≥ 21 | ≥ 18 | ≥ 13 | ≥ 12 |
| Average | 16–21 | 14–20 | 12–17 | 9–12 | 6–11 |
| Below average | 11–15 | 10–13 | 7–11 | 3–8 | 2–5 |
| Low | ≤ 10 | ≤ 9 | ≤ 6 | ≤ 2 | ≤ 1 |

ACSM's Guidelines for Exercise Testing and Prescription, 6th edition (based on data from the Canada Fitness Survey, 1981. Canadian Standardized Test of Fitness Operations Manual, 3rd edition, Ottawa: Fitness and Amateur Sports Canada, 1986).

After the walking test, Jackie and Frank moved to the football field sidelines to do the push-up test. Jackie went first. She warmed up with the appropriate stretches, and then asked Frank to check her position against the one in the photo. Frank counted as Jackie completed 13 push-ups, which, according to the muscular fitness norms table, indicate she is in the "Average" (yellow) category. After Jackie recorded her results on her personal fitness profile, she checked Frank's push-up position and counted for him as he did the test. Frank did 19 push-ups, which puts him in the "average" (yellow) category, too.

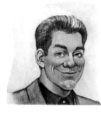

# Frank's Results:
# 19 Push-Ups

## Male Norms for the Push-Up Test (Number Completed)

| Rating | Age (years) | | | | |
| --- | --- | --- | --- | --- | --- |
| | 20–29 | 30–39 | 40–49 | 50–59 | 60–69 |
| Above average | ≥ 30 | ≥ 24 | ≥ 19 | ≥ 14 | ≥ 11 |
| Average | 24–29 | 19–23 | 13–18 | 10–13 | 9–10 |
| Below average | 18–23 | 14–18 | 10–12 | 7–9 | 6–7 |
| Low | ≤ 17 | ≤ 13 | ≤ 9 | ≤ 6 | ≤ 5 |

| Muscular Fitness | Push-Ups | 8/5 | Number: 19 | Average: Yellow |
| --- | --- | --- | --- | --- |
| | | | Number: | |
| | | | Numbe | |

## Sit-and-Reach Test

### Equipment

- Yardstick
- Adhesive tape

### Preparation

- Secure the yardstick to the floor by placing a 12-inch (30.5 cm) piece of tape across it at the 15-inch (38.1 cm) mark.
- Warm up, being sure to include the seated toe touch (page 116).

### Procedures

1. Position yourself on the floor with the yardstick between your legs (zero mark toward you) and the soles of your feet about 12 inches (30.5 cm) apart and even with the tape at the 15-inch (38.1 cm) mark.

2. Ask your friend to position his or her hands across your knees to gently hold them down when you stretch forward.

3. Place one hand on top of the other so that the middle fingers of each hand are even.

4. Gently lean forward along the yardstick, reaching as far as possible while exhaling and dropping the head between the arms. Hold the position for two seconds. Do not bounce or reach to the point of pain in the back of the legs or lower back, because this could cause an injury.

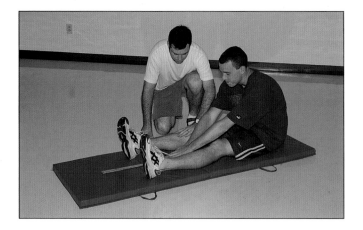

5. Note the distance reached.

6. Relax, then repeat the reach two more times.

7. Record your best score on your personal fitness profile.

## Determining Your Fitness Level

- Compare your best score to the standards in the following sit-and-reach table. Be sure to use the standards for your age and sex.

- Once you have determined your flexibility fitness level, record it on your personal fitness profile.

## Male Norms for the Sit-and-Reach Test (number of inches)

| Rating | Age (years) 18–25 | 26–35 | 36–45 | 46–55 | 56–65 | > 65 |
|---|---|---|---|---|---|---|
| Above average | ≥ 19 | ≥ 17 | ≥ 17 | ≥ 15 | ≥ 13 | ≥ 13 |
| Average | 17–18 | 15–16 | 15–16 | 13–14 | 11–12 | 10–12 |
| Below average | 14–16 | 13–14 | 13–14 | 10–12 | 9–10 | 8–9 |
| Low | ≤ 13 | ≤ 12 | ≤ 12 | ≤ 9 | ≤ 8 | ≤ 7 |

## Female Norms for the Sit-and-Reach Test (number of inches)

| Rating | Age (years) 18–25 | 26–35 | 36–45 | 46–55 | 56–65 | > 65 |
|---|---|---|---|---|---|---|
| Above average | ≥ 21 | ≥ 20 | ≥ 19 | ≥ 18 | ≥ 17 | ≥ 17 |
| Average | 19–20 | 19 | 17–18 | 16–17 | 15–16 | 15–16 |
| Below average | 17–18 | 16–18 | 15–16 | 14–15 | 13–14 | 13–14 |
| Low | ≤ 16 | ≤ 15 | ≤ 14 | ≤ 13 | ≤ 12 | ≤ 12 |

ACSM's Guidelines for Exercise Testing and Prescription, 6th edition, 2000 (Golding, L.A., Myers, C.R., Sinning, W.E., eds. Y's Way to Physical Fitness, 3rd edition, Champaign, IL: Human Kinetics, 1989).

Frank and Jackie walked to Jackie's house after they finished their push-up tests. Frank warmed up with the seated toe touch stretch as Jackie taped the yardstick to her kitchen floor. Frank looked at the photo and got into the proper position. Jackie held his knees down as he reached forward as far as he could three times, holding for two seconds each time. Frank recorded his best score—13 inches (33 centimeters)—on his fitness profile. He saw in the sit-and-reach table that a score of 13 for a 37-year-old man puts him in the blue "Below average" category. Jackie completed her warm-up while Frank was recording his score, and she was ready to begin. Jackie reached the farthest on the second of her three tries, and she recorded her score of 14 inches (35.5 centimeters)— "Below Average" (green on her personal fitness profile).

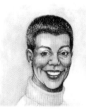

# Jackie's Results:
# 14 inches (35.5 cm)

## Female Norms for the Sit-and-Reach Test (number of inches)

| Rating | Age (years) | | | | | |
|---|---|---|---|---|---|---|
| | 18–25 | 26–35 | 36–45 | 46–55 | 56–65 | > 65 |
| Above average | ≥ 21 | ≥ 20 | ≥ 19 | ≥ 18 | ≥ 17 | ≥ 17 |
| Average | 19–20 | 19 | 17–18 | 16–17 | 15–16 | 15–16 |
| Below average | 17–18 | 16–18 | 15–16 | 14–15 | 13–14 | 13–14 |
| Low | ≤ 16 | ≤ 15 | ≤ 14 | ≤ 13 | ≤ 12 | ≤ 12 |

| Flexibility | Sit and Reach | 8/5 | Inches: 14 | Below avg: Green |
|---|---|---|---|---|
| | | | Inches: | |
| | | | Inc | |

## Body Mass Index and Waist-to-Hip Ratio

Appropriate amounts of both fat and lean tissue are necessary for optimal health. However, actually measuring the relative proportion of fat versus lean tissue in your body is very complex and can typically be done only in a laboratory set up for this kind of measurement. However, you can "estimate" your body composition using the Body Mass Index (BMI) or the Waist-to-Hip Ratio. These two procedures are used here to help you determine your body composition.

### Equipment

- Tape measure
- Scale to measure your weight

### Preparation

- Wear minimal clothes and remove your shoes.

### Procedures

1. Measure your weight on the scale.
2. Use the measuring tape to measure your height as you stand against a wall with your head, shoulders, buttocks, and heels against the wall.

3. Use the measuring tape to measure the circumference of your hips at the widest part of your buttocks and measure your waist at the smallest circumference of your natural waist, usually just above the navel (belly button). Measure at the end of a normal exhalation without pulling the tape tight.

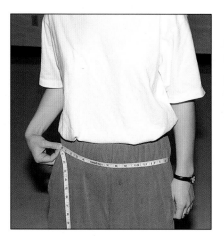 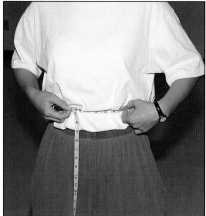

## Determining Your Fitness Level

### Body Mass Index

- Find your weight along the left side of the BMI chart, and draw a horizontal line across the graph.
- Find your height along the top of the chart, and draw a straight line down the graph.
- Read your BMI at the intersection of the two lines you have just drawn.

# Body Mass Index Chart

| Height (in.) | 49 | 51 | 53 | 55 | 57 | 59 | 61 | 63 | 65 | 67 | 69 | 71 | 73 | 75 | 77 | 79 | 81 | 83 |
|---|---|---|---|---|---|---|---|---|---|---|---|---|---|---|---|---|---|---|
| Weight (lb) | | | | | | | | | | | | | | | | | | |
| 66 | 19 | 18 | 16 | 15 | 14 | 13 | 12 | 12 | 11 | 10 | 10 | 9 | 9 | 8 | 8 | 8 | 7 | 7 |
| 70 | 20 | 19 | 18 | 16 | 15 | 14 | 13 | 13 | 12 | 11 | 10 | 10 | 9 | 9 | 8 | 8 | 8 | 7 |
| 75 | 22 | 20 | 19 | 17 | 16 | 15 | 14 | 13 | 12 | 12 | 11 | 10 | 10 | 9 | 9 | 9 | 8 | 8 |
| 79 | 23 | 21 | 20 | 18 | 17 | 16 | 15 | 14 | 13 | 12 | 12 | 11 | 11 | 10 | 9 | 9 | 9 | 8 |
| 84 | 24 | 22 | 21 | 19 | 18 | 17 | 16 | 15 | 14 | 13 | 12 | 12 | 11 | 11 | 10 | 10 | 9 | 9 |
| 88 | 26 | 24 | 22 | 20 | 19 | 18 | 17 | 16 | 15 | 14 | 13 | 12 | 12 | 11 | 11 | 10 | 10 | 9 |
| 92 | 27 | 25 | 23 | 21 | 20 | 19 | 17 | 16 | 15 | 15 | 14 | 13 | 12 | 12 | 11 | 11 | 10 | 10 |
| 97 | 28 | 26 | 24 | 22 | 21 | 20 | 18 | 17 | 16 | 15 | 14 | 14 | 13 | 12 | 12 | 11 | 10 | 10 |
| 101 | 29 | 27 | 25 | 23 | 22 | 20 | 19 | 18 | 17 | 16 | 15 | 14 | 13 | 13 | 12 | 12 | 11 | 10 |
| 106 | 31 | 28 | 26 | 24 | 23 | 21 | 20 | 19 | 18 | 17 | 16 | 15 | 14 | 13 | 13 | 12 | 11 | 11 |
| 110 | 32 | 30 | 27 | 26 | 24 | 22 | 21 | 20 | 18 | 17 | 16 | 15 | 15 | 14 | 13 | 13 | 11 | 11 |
| 114 | 33 | 31 | 29 | 27 | 25 | 23 | 22 | 20 | 19 | 18 | 17 | 16 | 15 | 14 | 14 | 13 | 12 | 12 |
| 119 | 35 | 32 | 30 | 28 | 26 | 24 | 22 | 21 | 20 | 19 | 18 | 17 | 16 | 15 | 14 | 14 | 13 | 12 |
| 123 | 36 | 33 | 31 | 29 | 27 | 25 | 23 | 22 | 21 | 19 | 18 | 17 | 16 | 16 | 15 | 14 | 13 | 13 |
| 128 | 37 | 34 | 32 | 30 | 28 | 26 | 24 | 23 | 21 | 20 | 19 | 18 | 17 | 16 | 15 | 15 | 14 | 13 |
| 132 | 38 | 36 | 33 | 31 | 29 | 27 | 25 | 23 | 22 | 21 | 20 | 19 | 18 | 17 | 16 | 15 | 14 | 14 |
| 136 | 40 | 37 | 34 | 32 | 29 | 28 | 26 | 24 | 23 | 21 | 20 | 19 | 18 | 17 | 16 | 16 | 15 | 14 |
| 141 | 41 | 38 | 35 | 33 | 30 | 28 | 27 | 25 | 24 | 22 | 21 | 20 | 19 | 18 | 17 | 16 | 15 | 15 |
| 145 | 42 | 39 | 36 | 34 | 31 | 29 | 27 | 26 | 24 | 23 | 22 | 20 | 19 | 18 | 17 | 17 | 16 | 15 |
| 150 | 44 | 40 | 37 | 35 | 32 | 30 | 28 | 27 | 25 | 24 | 22 | 21 | 20 | 19 | 18 | 17 | 16 | 15 |
| 154 | 45 | 41 | 38 | 36 | 33 | 31 | 29 | 27 | 26 | 24 | 23 | 22 | 20 | 19 | 18 | 18 | 17 | 16 |
| 158 | 46 | 43 | 40 | 37 | 34 | 32 | 30 | 28 | 26 | 25 | 24 | 22 | 21 | 20 | 19 | 18 | 17 | 16 |
| 163 | 47 | 44 | 41 | 38 | 35 | 33 | 31 | 29 | 27 | 26 | 24 | 23 | 22 | 20 | 19 | 19 | 18 | 17 |
| 167 | 49 | 45 | 42 | 39 | 36 | 34 | 32 | 30 | 28 | 26 | 25 | 23 | 22 | 21 | 20 | 19 | 18 | 17 |
| 172 | 50 | 46 | 43 | 40 | 37 | 35 | 32 | 30 | 29 | 27 | 25 | 24 | 23 | 22 | 21 | 20 | 19 | 18 |
| 176 | 51 | 47 | 44 | 41 | 38 | 36 | 33 | 31 | 29 | 28 | 26 | 25 | 23 | 22 | 21 | 20 | 19 | 18 |
| 180 | 52 | 49 | 45 | 42 | 39 | 36 | 34 | 32 | 30 | 28 | 27 | 25 | 24 | 23 | 22 | 21 | 20 | 19 |
| 185 | 54 | 50 | 46 | 43 | 40 | 37 | 35 | 33 | 31 | 29 | 27 | 26 | 25 | 23 | 22 | 21 | 20 | 19 |
| 189 | 55 | 51 | 47 | 44 | 41 | 38 | 36 | 34 | 32 | 30 | 28 | 27 | 25 | 24 | 23 | 22 | 20 | 20 |
| 194 | 56 | 52 | 48 | 45 | 42 | 39 | 37 | 34 | 32 | 30 | 29 | 27 | 26 | 24 | 23 | 22 | 21 | 20 |
| 198 | 58 | 53 | 49 | 46 | 43 | 40 | 37 | 35 | 33 | 31 | 29 | 28 | 26 | 25 | 24 | 23 | 21 | 20 |
| 202 | 59 | 54 | 50 | 47 | 44 | 41 | 38 | 36 | 34 | 32 | 30 | 28 | 27 | 25 | 24 | 23 | 22 | 21 |
| 207 | 60 | 56 | 52 | 48 | 45 | 42 | 39 | 37 | 35 | 33 | 31 | 29 | 27 | 26 | 25 | 24 | 22 | 21 |
| 211 | 61 | 57 | 53 | 49 | 46 | 43 | 40 | 38 | 35 | 33 | 31 | 30 | 28 | 27 | 25 | 24 | 23 | 22 |
| 216 | 63 | 58 | 54 | 50 | 47 | 44 | 41 | 38 | 36 | 34 | 32 | 30 | 29 | 27 | 26 | 25 | 23 | 22 |
| 220 | 64 | 59 | 55 | 51 | 48 | 44 | 42 | 39 | 37 | 35 | 33 | 31 | 29 | 28 | 26 | 25 | 24 | 23 |
| 224 | 65 | 60 | 56 | 52 | 49 | 45 | 42 | 40 | 37 | 35 | 33 | 31 | 30 | 28 | 27 | 26 | 24 | 23 |
| 229 | 67 | 62 | 57 | 53 | 49 | 46 | 43 | 41 | 38 | 36 | 34 | 32 | 30 | 29 | 27 | 26 | 25 | 24 |
| 233 | 68 | 63 | 58 | 54 | 50 | 47 | 44 | 41 | 39 | 37 | 35 | 33 | 31 | 29 | 28 | 27 | 25 | 24 |
| 238 | 69 | 64 | 59 | 55 | 51 | 48 | 45 | 42 | 40 | 37 | 35 | 33 | 32 | 30 | 28 | 27 | 26 | 24 |
| 242 | 70 | 65 | 60 | 56 | 52 | 49 | 46 | 43 | 40 | 38 | 36 | 34 | 32 | 30 | 29 | 28 | 26 | 25 |
| 246 | 72 | 66 | 61 | 57 | 53 | 50 | 47 | 44 | 41 | 39 | 37 | 35 | 33 | 31 | 29 | 28 | 27 | 25 |
| 251 | 73 | 67 | 63 | 58 | 54 | 51 | 47 | 45 | 42 | 39 | 37 | 35 | 33 | 32 | 30 | 29 | 27 | 26 |
| 255 | 74 | 69 | 64 | 59 | 55 | 52 | 48 | 45 | 43 | 40 | 38 | 36 | 34 | 32 | 31 | 29 | 28 | 26 |
| 260 | 76 | 70 | 65 | 60 | 56 | 52 | 49 | 46 | 43 | 41 | 39 | 36 | 34 | 33 | 31 | 30 | 28 | 27 |
| 264 | 77 | 71 | 66 | 61 | 57 | 53 | 50 | 47 | 44 | 42 | 39 | 37 | 35 | 33 | 32 | 30 | 29 | 27 |
| 268 | 78 | 72 | 67 | 62 | 58 | 54 | 51 | 48 | 45 | 42 | 40 | 38 | 36 | 34 | 32 | 31 | 29 | 28 |
| 273 | 79 | 73 | 68 | 63 | 59 | 55 | 52 | 48 | 46 | 43 | 40 | 38 | 36 | 34 | 33 | 31 | 30 | 28 |
| 277 | 81 | 75 | 69 | 64 | 60 | 56 | 52 | 49 | 46 | 44 | 41 | 39 | 37 | 35 | 33 | 32 | 30 | 29 |
| 282 | 82 | 76 | 70 | 65 | 61 | 57 | 53 | 50 | 47 | 44 | 42 | 40 | 37 | 35 | 34 | 32 | 30 | 29 |
| 286 | 83 | 77 | 71 | 66 | 62 | 58 | 54 | 51 | 48 | 45 | 42 | 40 | 38 | 36 | 34 | 33 | 31 | 29 |
| 290 | 84 | 78 | 72 | 67 | 63 | 59 | 55 | 52 | 48 | 46 | 43 | 41 | 39 | 37 | 35 | 33 | 31 | 30 |
| 295 | 86 | 79 | 74 | 68 | 64 | 60 | 56 | 52 | 49 | 46 | 44 | 41 | 39 | 37 | 35 | 34 | 32 | 30 |
| 299 | 87 | 80 | 75 | 69 | 65 | 60 | 57 | 53 | 50 | 47 | 44 | 42 | 40 | 38 | 36 | 34 | 32 | 31 |
| 304 | 88 | 82 | 76 | 70 | 66 | 61 | 57 | 54 | 51 | 48 | 45 | 43 | 40 | 38 | 36 | 35 | 33 | 31 |
| 308 | 90 | 83 | 77 | 71 | 67 | 62 | 58 | 55 | 51 | 48 | 46 | 43 | 41 | 39 | 37 | 35 | 33 | 32 |
| 312 | 91 | 84 | 78 | 72 | 68 | 63 | 59 | 55 | 52 | 49 | 46 | 44 | 41 | 39 | 37 | 36 | 34 | 32 |

Note: Categories are based on values published by the Panel on Energy, Obesity, and Body Weight Standards, 1987, *American Journal of Clinical Nutrition, 45*, p. 1035.

Jackie brought her scales from her bathroom to the kitchen so she and Frank could do the body composition tests. Both removed their shoes and measured each other as each stood against the kitchen wall. They moved to the scales and weighed each other. Frank recorded his height and weight. He measured 5 feet, 11 inches (1.8 meters) tall and weighed 178 pounds (80.8 kilograms). Jackie recorded her results: 5 feet, 6 inches (1.68 meters), and 157 pounds (71.2 kilograms). According to the BMI chart, Frank's height of 71 inches intersects with his 178-pound weight at the number 25. Jackie's height and weight of 66 inches and 157 pounds give her a BMI score between 24 and 26.

# Jackie's Results:
# 66 inches (1.68 m),
# 157 pounds (71.2 kg)

| Height (in.) | 49 | 51 | 53 | 55 | 57 | 59 | 61 | 63 | 65 | 67 | 69 | 71 | 73 | 75 | 77 | 79 | 81 | 83 |
|---|---|---|---|---|---|---|---|---|---|---|---|---|---|---|---|---|---|---|
| Weight (lb) | | | | | | | | | | | | | | | | | | |
| 66 | 19 | 18 | 16 | 15 | 14 | 13 | 12 | 12 | 11 | 10 | 10 | 9 | 9 | 8 | 8 | 8 | 7 | 7 |
| 70 | 20 | 19 | 18 | 16 | 15 | 14 | 13 | 13 | 12 | 11 | 10 | 10 | 9 | 9 | 8 | 8 | 8 | 7 |
| 75 | 22 | 20 | 19 | 17 | 16 | 15 | 14 | 13 | 12 | 12 | 11 | 10 | 10 | 9 | 9 | 9 | 8 | 8 |
| 79 | 23 | 21 | 20 | 18 | 17 | 16 | 15 | 14 | 13 | 12 | 12 | 11 | 11 | 10 | 9 | 9 | 9 | 8 |
| 84 | 24 | 22 | 21 | 19 | 18 | 17 | 16 | 15 | 14 | 13 | 12 | 12 | 11 | 11 | 10 | 10 | 9 | 9 |
| 88 | 26 | 24 | 22 | 20 | 19 | 18 | 17 | 16 | 15 | 14 | 13 | 12 | 12 | 11 | 11 | 10 | 10 | 9 |
| 92 | 27 | 25 | 23 | 21 | 20 | 19 | 17 | 16 | 15 | 15 | 14 | 13 | 12 | 12 | 11 | 11 | 10 | 10 |
| 97 | 28 | 26 | 24 | 22 | 21 | 20 | 18 | 17 | 16 | 15 | 14 | 14 | 13 | 12 | 12 | 11 | 10 | 10 |
| 101 | 29 | 27 | 25 | 23 | 22 | 20 | 19 | 18 | 17 | 16 | 15 | 14 | 13 | 13 | 12 | 12 | 11 | 10 |
| 106 | 31 | 28 | 26 | 24 | 23 | 21 | 20 | 19 | 18 | 17 | 16 | 15 | 14 | 13 | 13 | 12 | 11 | 11 |
| 110 | 32 | 30 | 27 | 26 | 24 | 22 | 21 | 20 | 18 | 17 | 16 | 15 | 15 | 14 | 13 | 13 | 11 | 11 |
| 114 | 33 | 31 | 29 | 27 | 25 | 23 | 22 | 20 | 19 | 18 | 17 | 16 | 15 | 14 | 14 | 13 | 12 | 12 |
| 119 | 35 | 32 | 30 | 28 | 26 | 24 | 22 | 21 | 20 | 19 | 18 | 17 | 16 | 15 | 14 | 14 | 13 | 12 |
| 123 | 36 | 33 | 31 | 29 | 27 | 25 | 23 | 22 | 21 | 19 | 18 | 17 | 16 | 16 | 15 | 14 | 13 | 13 |
| 128 | 37 | 34 | 32 | 30 | 28 | 26 | 24 | 23 | 21 | 20 | 19 | 18 | 17 | 16 | 15 | 15 | 14 | 13 |
| 132 | 38 | 36 | 33 | 31 | 29 | 27 | 25 | 23 | 22 | 21 | 20 | 19 | 18 | 17 | 16 | 15 | 14 | 14 |
| 136 | 40 | 37 | 34 | 32 | 29 | 28 | 26 | 24 | 23 | 21 | 20 | 19 | 18 | 17 | 16 | 16 | 15 | 14 |
| 141 | 41 | 38 | 35 | 33 | 30 | 28 | 27 | 25 | 24 | 22 | 21 | 20 | 19 | 18 | 17 | 16 | 15 | 15 |
| 145 | 42 | 39 | 36 | 34 | 31 | 29 | 27 | 26 | 24 | 23 | 22 | 20 | 19 | 18 | 17 | 17 | 16 | 15 |
| 150 | 44 | 40 | 37 | 35 | 32 | 30 | 28 | 27 | 25 | 24 | 22 | 21 | 20 | 19 | 18 | 17 | 16 | |
| 154 | 45 | 41 | 38 | 36 | 33 | 31 | 29 | 27 | 26 | 24 | 23 | 22 | 20 | 19 | 18 | 18 | 1 | |
| 158 | 46 | 43 | 40 | 37 | 34 | 32 | 30 | 28 | 26 | 25 | 24 | 22 | 21 | 20 | 19 | 18 | | |
| 163 | 47 | 44 | 41 | 38 | 35 | 33 | 31 | 29 | 27 | 26 | 24 | 23 | 22 | | | | | |
| 167 | 49 | 45 | 42 | 39 | 36 | 34 | 32 | 30 | 28 | 26 | 25 | 23 | | | | | | |
| 172 | 50 | 46 | 43 | 40 | 37 | 35 | 32 | 30 | 29 | 27 | | | | | | | | |
| 176 | 51 | 47 | 44 | 41 | 38 | | | | | | | | | | | | | |
| 180 | 52 | 49 | 45 | | | | | | | | | | | | | | | |

# Waist-to-Hip Ratio

- Divide your waist measurement by your hip measurement.
- Record your waist-to-hip ratio on the personal fitness profile.

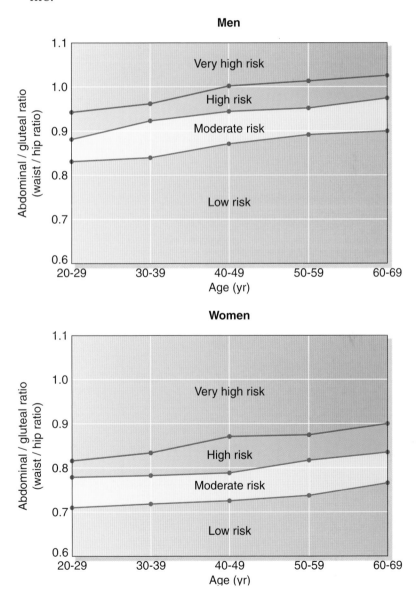

Reprinted by permission of *The Western Journal of Medicine* (G.A. Bray and D.S. Gray, Obesity: Part I—Pathogenesis, 1988, volume 149, pages 429–441).

# Body Composition Fitness Level

Use the body composition table to determine your body composition fitness level. Record it on your personal fitness profile.

| BMI category | W/H category | Fitness level |
|---|---|---|
| Greater than 30 | Very high risk | Green |
| | High risk | Green |
| | Moderate risk | Green |
| | Low risk | Green |
| 26-30 | Very high risk | Green |
| | High risk | Green |
| | Moderate risk | Yellow |
| | Low risk | Yellow |
| 19-25 | Very high risk | Yellow |
| | High risk | Yellow |
| | Moderate risk | Red |
| | Low risk | Red |
| Less than 19 | Very high risk | Blue |
| | High risk | Blue |
| | Moderate risk | Blue |
| | Low risk | Blue |

Next, Jackie and Frank measured each other's hips and waists, using the photos as a guide for positioning the tape measure. Frank's hips measured 40 inches (101.6 centimeters) and his waist was 38 inches (96.52 centimeters). Using a calculator to divide 38 by 40, Frank found his waist-to-hip ratio was 0.95, which puts him in the "High risk" category. Jackie's waist was 33 inches (83.8 centimeters), and her hips were 42 inches (106.7 centimeters). Jackie's waist-to-hip ratio of 0.79 puts her in the "Moderate risk" category.

Jackie and Frank used the body composition fitness level chart to find their body composition fitness levels. Jackie, with a BMI score of approximately 25 and a waist-to-hip ratio that is in the "Moderate risk" category, is at the red level. Frank, with a BMI score of 25 and a waist-to-hip ratio in the "High risk" category, is at the yellow level. Jackie and Frank recorded their results on the personal fitness profile.

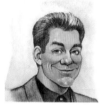

# Frank's Results:
# Waist: 38 inches (96.52 cm)
# Hips: 40 inches (101.6 cm)

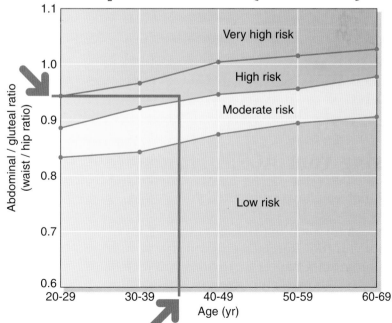

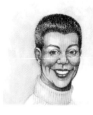

# Jackie's Results: Moderate risk fitness level

| BMI category | W/H category | Fitness level |
|:---:|:---:|:---:|
| 26-30 | Very high risk | Green |
| | High risk | Green |
| | Moderate risk | Yellow |
| | Low risk | Yellow |
| (19-25) | Very high risk | Yellow |
| | High risk | Yellow |
| | (Moderate risk) | Red |
| | Low risk | Red |

| Body Composition | Body Mass Index and Waist-to-Hip Ratio | 8/5 | BMI: 25 W/H: .79 | Moderate Risk: Red |
|---|---|---|---|---|
| | | | BMI: W/H: | |
| | | | BMI: | |

# Using Your ACSM Fitness Test Results

Now that you have completed your ACSM Fitness Test, you are ready to begin the exercises designed especially for your level of fitness for each of the four components of fitness. Chapter 5 shows you the exercises you will use in your own personal fitness program. Chapter 6 provides you with daily activity charts to let you know which exercises to perform to ensure safe, gradual improvement in your personal fitness.

# ACSM Personal Fitness Profile
## for

### Jackie

Your Name

| Fitness Component | Test | Date | Scores | Fitness Level & Color |
|---|---|---|---|---|
| Aerobic Fitness | Rockport 1-Mile Walk (1.6 km) | 8/5 | Time: 18:15 HR: 132 bpm | Below avg: Green |
| | | | Time: HR: | |
| | | | Time: HR: | |
| | | | Time: HR: | |
| Muscular Fitness | Push-Ups | 8/5 | Number: 13 | Average: Yellow |
| | | | Number: | |
| | | | Number: | |
| | | | Number: | |
| Flexibility | Sit and Reach | 8/5 | Inches: 13 | Below avg: Green |
| | | | Inches: | |
| | | | Inches: | |
| | | | Inches: | |
| Body Composition | Body Mass Index and Waist-to-Hip Ratio | 8/5 | BMI: 25 W/H: .79 | Moderate Risk: Red |
| | | | BMI: W/H: | |
| | | | BMI: W/H: | |
| | | | BMI: W/H: | |

CHAPTER

# 5

# Beginning Exercises

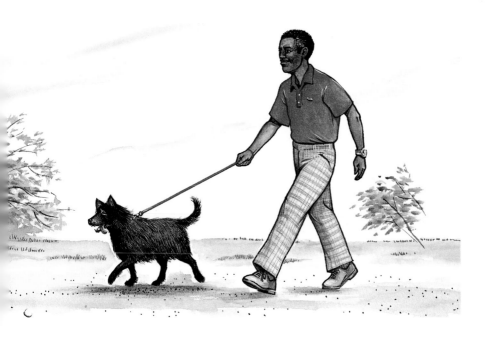

**N**ow that you have made the commitment to begin a sustained program for a healthier future and you have done all the necessary assessments found in the ACSM Fitness Test, it is time to start to build an exercise program that will address your specific goals. One of the best ways to start to increase your daily physical activity is to become more aware of the opportunities in your daily life. You can walk your dog, play ball with your grandchildren, mow the lawn, or garden. You can take the stairs more often (rather than wait for an elevator) or park the car farther away from a store entrance.

This chapter will help you include specific exercises that will enable you to reach your goals and stay committed to the program. It presents safe, effective exercises that will become part of your individualized fitness program. Exercises for all fitness components—aerobic fitness, muscular fitness, flexibility, and body composition—are included. In this chapter, we show you the exercises and provide hints on how to get the greatest benefit from the exercise program. In chapter 6, we help you put the exercises together in programs designed for your personal fitness level and goals established when you took the ACSM Fitness Test.

The exercises in this chapter allow you to gradually increase your fitness. Exercise does not have to hurt to be effective. The old saying "No pain, no gain," is not true. Research has demonstrated that you do not have to exercise at high intensities to get positive health benefits. In fact, we will show you how to reach your goals using only moderately intense exercise.

Here are some general guidelines to follow when exercising for health and fitness:

• Wear loose, comfortable clothing and sturdy athletic shoes (a good investment).

• Warm up and cool down after each exercise session.

• Exercise at an intensity high enough that you feel invigorated but not exhausted. When your exercise intensity is appropriate, your breathing rate increases, but you are still able to carry on a conversation.

• Take special care when exercising in hot and humid weather:

a. Slow down your walk or other activity.

b. Exercise early in the morning or later in the evening, or in air conditioning.

c. Drink plenty of water before, during, and after exercise.

d. Cool down for a longer period of time.

• Because exercise is only a benefit if you are feeling well, do not try to exercise when you have a cold, the flu, or another illness. Wait until you are feeling better to resume your program.

• If you miss your exercise sessions for more than a week, make sure to start out again slowly. Resume your program by repeating the exercises you did a few days before your last workout, then progress normally from that new point. Following this advice will reduce your chances of injury.

# Aerobic Fitness

The definition of *aerobic fitness* is the body's increased ability to take in and use oxygen to produce energy. A higher level of aerobic fitness will give you more endurance and will increase your ability to work at a higher level over a longer period of time.

Many activities can improve aerobic fitness, including walking, biking, dancing, skating, and rowing, all of which keep your whole body moving in a continuous, rhythmic manner. The ACSM Fitness Program uses walking as an example of an aerobic fitness activity. Walking is one of the better physical activities. It can be done almost anywhere and requires no special equipment. Walking puts very little strain on the joints and involves most of the major muscle groups. It can be done alone or with a group, at whatever pace is comfortable. For all these reasons, walking is one of the most popular forms of exercise. In chapter 6, we give specific daily walking goals as part of your fitness program.

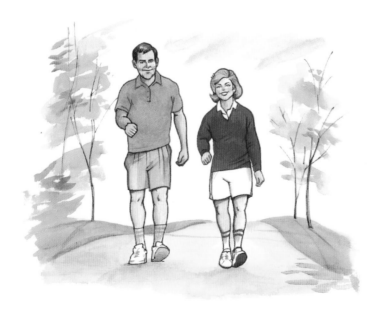

If, for some reason, you cannot or do not want to walk as part of your individualized fitness program, you can substitute any other aerobic activity (such as cycling on an exercise bike, outdoor cycling, dancing, or skating). Simply follow the same time guidelines that we have given for our example of walking.

# Muscular Fitness

Muscular fitness is the increased strength and endurance of your muscles. A higher level of muscular strength and endurance allows you to work longer before you get tired; thus strength and endurance is related to aerobic fitness. The best way to ensure that you work all major muscle groups of the body is to combine a variety of exercises. We have arranged these exercises by muscle groups for you. Your own personal fitness program will include some, but not all, of the exercises. The programs we develop for you in chapter 6 use these exercises. The text in parentheses next to the name of each exercise tells you in what program level the exercise is used. At the end of the muscular fitness exercise section, we have included some additional exercises that you can use if you want to add a little variety to your muscular fitness program.

Many of the muscular fitness exercises can be done using hand or leg weights. Plastic milk, water, or detergent jugs partially filled with sand or water make good weights if you do not want to purchase dumbbells or barbells. The amount of sand or water can be adjusted as your fitness progresses. When using weights, be sure to make all movements slowly and deliberately. If you experience any pain in any of your joints when using weights, reduce the amount of weight, or stop using them completely.

In the past, many women thought they should avoid exercising with weights because they did not want to develop large, bulky muscles. Most women, however, have a genetic makeup that prevents them from developing the large muscles that many men develop when using weights. Our advice for women who want to gain muscular strength and endurance is to go ahead and use weights, then check out the benefits.

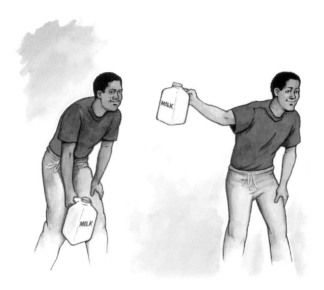

Remember these training principles as you complete your muscular fitness exercises:

- Complete all movements slowly and with complete control.
- Maintain normal breathing patterns throughout the exercise.
- Stop any exercise that causes pain.
- Stretch each muscle group after your workout.

# Body Composition

The ratio of a body's fat tissue to its lean tissue (muscles, bones, organs) is known as body composition (review chapter 2). The best way to achieve a healthy body composition is to burn Calories through regular exercise while using resistance exercise to build lean tissue. If losing body fat is your goal, complete your aerobic fitness program four to six days per week. That, along with a diet low in fat and total calories, will help you to lose the most fat. Most important, make an effort to increase the total amount of activity in your daily life.

# ARMS AND SHOULDERS

## ▼ Wall Push-Up (Level 1)

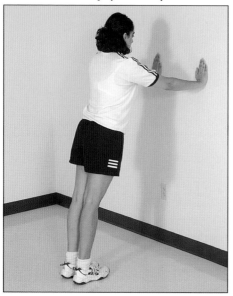

Push your body away from the wall . . .

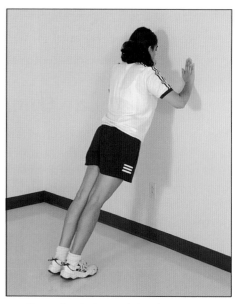

. . . then slowly lower it back.

## ▼ Chair Push-Up (Level 2)

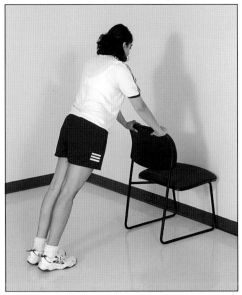

Position the chair against a wall so it won't slide and fully extend your arms.

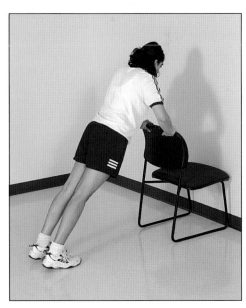

Lower your body toward the chair.

### ▼ Knee Push-Up (Level 3)

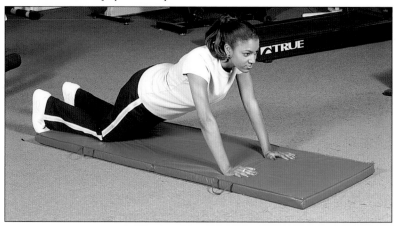

Keep your back straight, fully extend
your arms, then lower your body to the
floor.

### ▼ Toe Push-Up (Level 4)

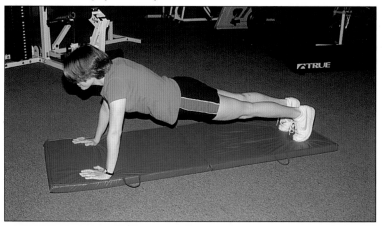

Keep your back straight, fully
extend your arms, then lower your
body to the floor.

## ▼ Single-Arm Row (Levels 1, 2, 3)

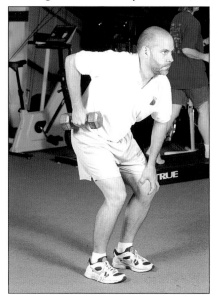 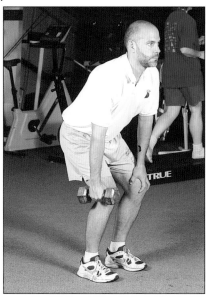

Pull the weight toward your shoulder . . .     . . . then ease it toward the floor.

## ▼ Biceps Curl (Level 4)

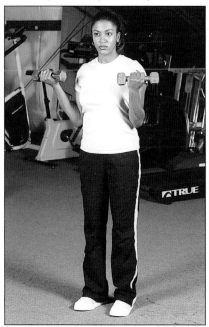 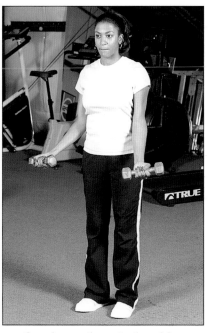

Bending at the elbow, lift the weights toward your shoulder . . .     . . . then lower them to the side without fully extending your arms.

### ▼ Reverse Fly (Level 4)

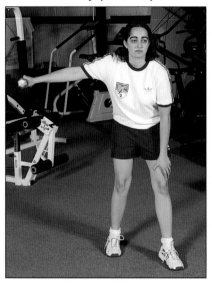
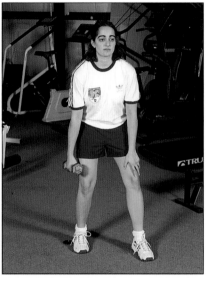

Use your shoulder and upper back muscles to lift the weight up and out.

Slowly lower the weight toward the floor. Keep your back straight and your neck relaxed.

## LEGS AND HIPS

### ▼ Seated Lower-Leg Lift (Level 1)

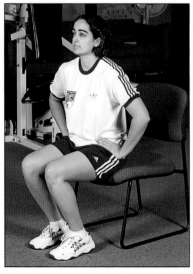
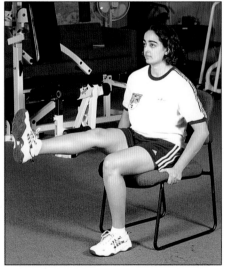

Sit comfortably in a chair.

Keep your thigh on the chair and straighten your leg without locking your knee.

## ▼ Seated Straight-Leg Lift (Level 2)

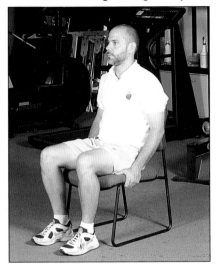

Sit comfortably.

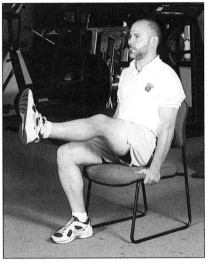

Straighten your leg and lift it off the chair, but not to full extension.

## ▼ Stair Step (Level 3)

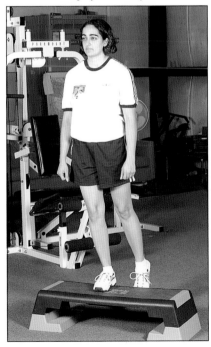

Step up to a straight-leg position.

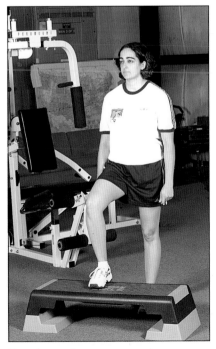

Bend your knee to step down.

## ▼ Chair Squat (Level 4)

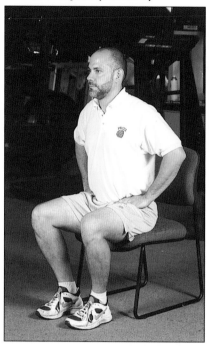

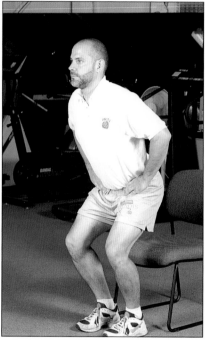

Sit at the edge of a chair and place your heels under the seat.

Stand up without leaning forward, keeping your hands on your hips. Do not fully extend your knees. Slowly return to the sitting position.

## ▼ Toe Raise (Levels 2, 4)

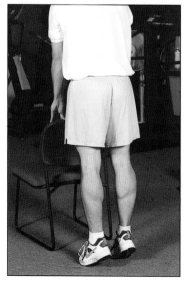

Use the back of a chair for stability; raise up on your toes, then lower your heels to the floor.

# ABDOMINALS

## ▼ Neck Curl-Up (Level 1)

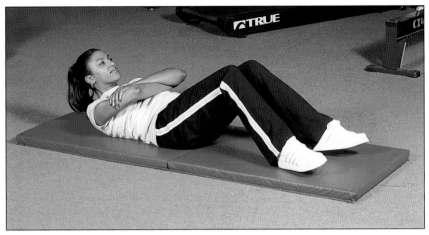

Keep your arms crossed and lift your head from the floor. Keep your lower back flat on the floor.

## ▼ Shoulder Curl-Up (Level 2)

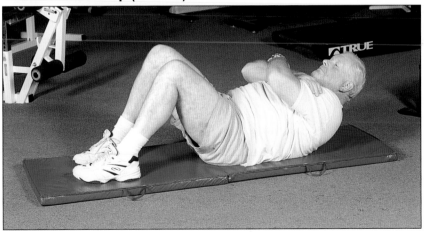

Keep your arms crossed and lift only the tops of your shoulders off the floor. Keep your lower back flat on the floor.

## ▼ Straight-Arm Curl-Up (Level 3)

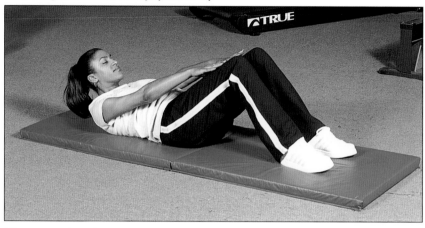

Place your hands on your thighs and lift your shoulders off the floor, sliding your hands toward your knees. Keep your head and neck relaxed.

## ▼ Crossed-Arm Curl-Up (Level 4)

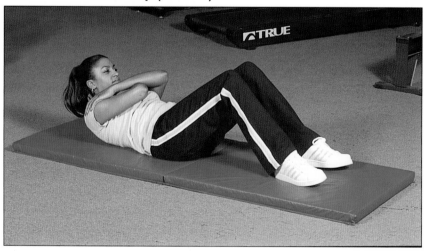

Cross your arms; keep your head and neck relaxed with a space between your chin and chest as you lift your shoulders off the floor.

# BACK

## ▼ Prone Neck Lift (Level 2)

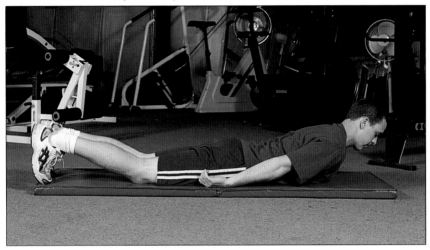

Slowly lift your forehead off the floor, keeping your neck straight.

## ▼ Prone Single-Leg Lift (Level 3)

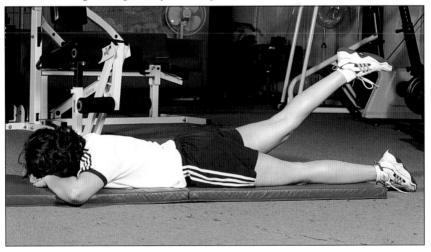

Slowly lift one leg from the hip, then switch legs, keeping your head on your hands.

### ▼ Prone Head- and Leg-Lift (Level 4)

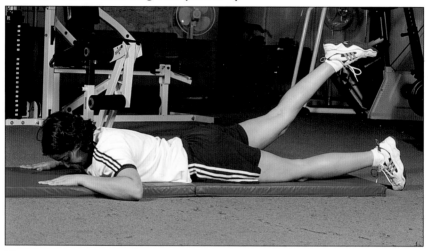

Keep your neck straight as you lift your forehead and one leg off the floor.

## ADDITIONAL EXERCISES

### ▼ Triceps Press (Arms)

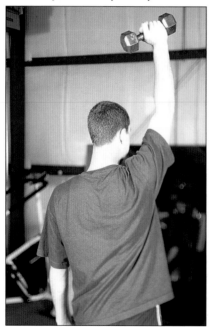 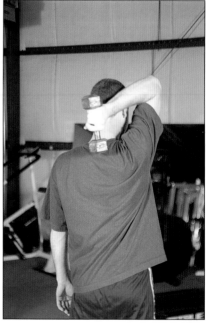

Keep your elbow high.

Lift and lower weight behind your head.

# ▼ Lateral Raise (Shoulders)

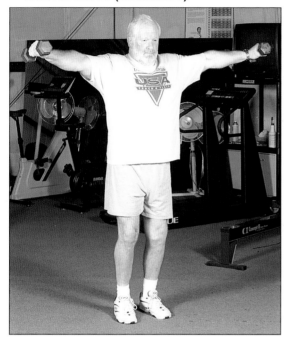

Keep your elbows slightly bent as you lift until your arms are parallel to the ground.

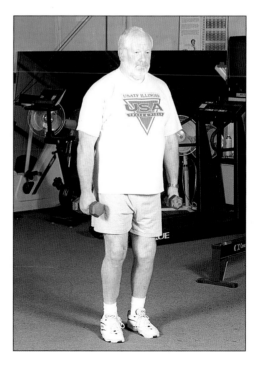

Lower the weights to your sides.

### ▼ Shrug (Shoulders and Upper Back)

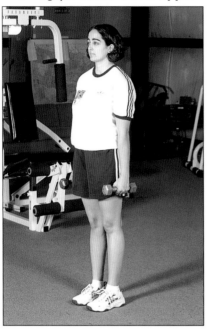 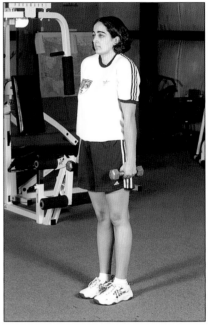

Keep your arms straight and your shoulders relaxed.

Lift your shoulders toward your ears.

### ▼ Inner-Leg Lift (Legs)

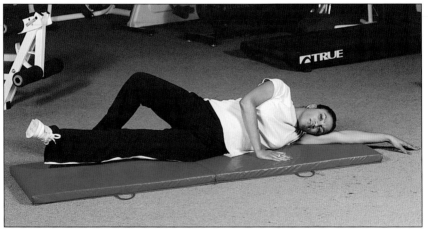

Lift your lower leg off the floor, keeping opposite leg stationary.

## ▼ Outer-Leg Lift (Legs)

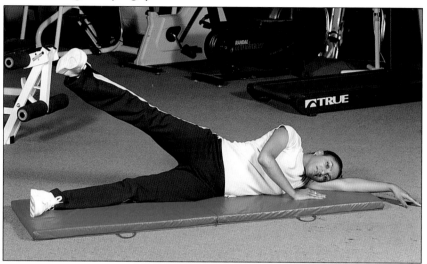

Raise your upper leg 16 to 20 inches (40.6 to 50.8 cm) off the floor.

| Exercises to Avoid | |
| --- | --- |
| Deep knee bend | Strains knees |
| Jumping jacks | Places strain on outside of knee |
| Full sit-up | Not effective in conditioning abdominals |
| Straight leg sit-up | May strain lower back |
| Double leg lift | Main strain lower back |
| Donkey kick | Hyperextends back |
| Bicycle | Places stress on neck and back |
| Squat thrust | Places strain on back and knees |

| Exercises to Avoid | |
|---|---|
| Standing toe touch | May strain lower back |
| Hurdler stretch | Puts strain on bent knee |
| Hyperextending or overrounding the back | Puts stress on neck and lower back |
| Full neck circle | Hyperextends the neck |
| Backbend | Ineffective in stretching stomach muscles |

# Flexibility

Flexibility is the ability to bend joints and stretch muscles through a full range of motion. This ability requires that the muscles around your joints be stretched safely and regularly. Every group of muscles in your body can be stretched without causing injury to your joints. A safe stretch is one that is gentle and relaxing: Move just until you can feel the muscle stretch. Hold the position for 10 to 20 seconds; then relax and repeat the stretch. If a stretch hurts, stop doing it. Pain is a signal from your body that something is wrong. Listen to your body and you will safely improve your flexibility.

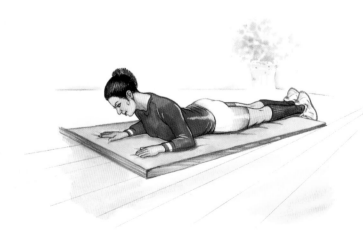

# NECK

### ▼ Head Tilt (Levels 1, 3, 4)

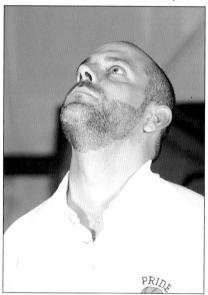 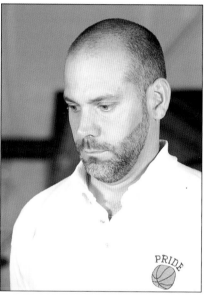

Tilt your head back and forth.

Bend where your head meets your neck, not from the lower neck.

### ▼ Head Turn (Levels 2, 4)

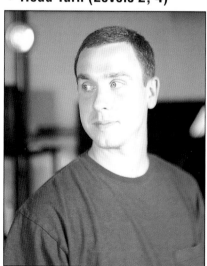

Turn your head slowly to look over one shoulder then the other.

## ▼ Head Lean

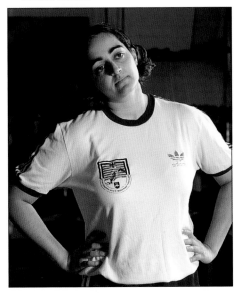

Keep your shoulders relaxed; lean your head toward one shoulder then the other.

# ARMS AND SHOULDERS

## ▼ Shoulder Rolls (All Levels)

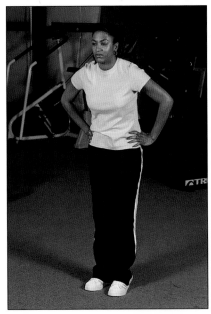

Place your hands on your hips.

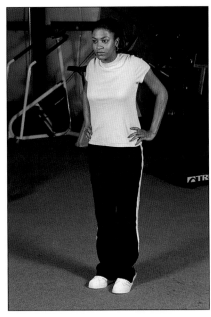

Rotate your shoulders backward, then forward.

## ▼ Shoulder Stretch (Level 2)

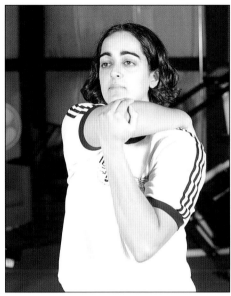

Use your left arm to gently pull the right elbow across your chest and vice versa.

## ▼ Arm Circles

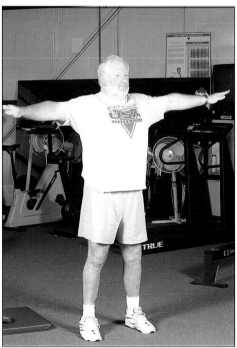

Slowly circle your arms from the shoulder.

# CHEST AND BACK

## ▼ Chest Stretch (All Levels)

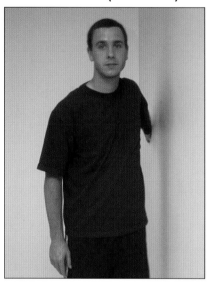

Place your outstretched arm against a wall, then turn away.

## ▼ Standing Cat Stretch (All Levels)

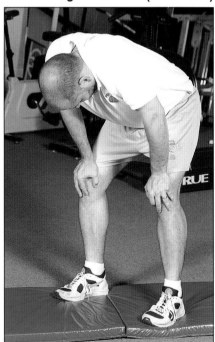

Round your back, then straighten it while leaning on your thighs, keeping your head stationary.

## ▼ Side Reach (All Levels)

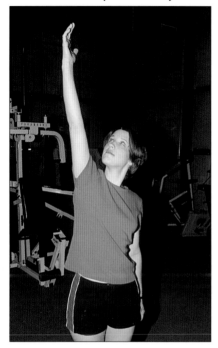

Reach up; do not bend over.

## ▼ Shoulder Turn (Level 3)

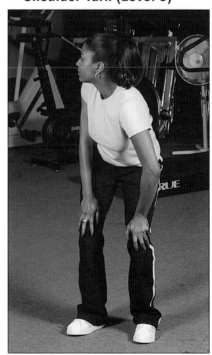

Place your hands on your knees and slowly turn the upper body to the left then to the right

## ▼ Long Lying Stretch (All Levels)

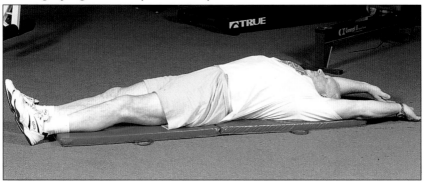

Press your lower back to the floor as you reach overhead.

## ▼ Single-Knee to Chest Stretch (Levels 2, 4)

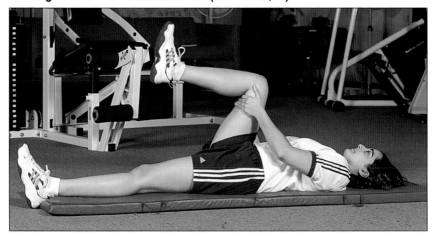

Place both hands on the back of the knee and draw it to the chest, keeping the other leg in contact with the ground.

### ▼ Double-Knee to Chest Stretch (Levels 3, 4)

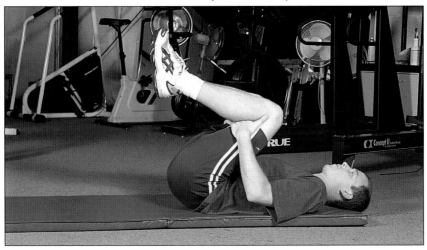

Place both hands on the back of both knees and draw them to the chest.

## LEGS AND HIPS

### ▼ Wall Lean (All Levels)

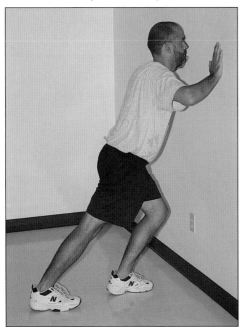

Keep your back heel on the ground with your foot turned slightly inward.

## ▼ Quadriceps Stretch (All Levels)

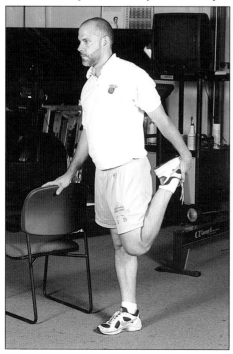

Grasp your foot and pull it up toward the buttocks, keeping your knee pointing toward the ground.

## ▼ Seated Toe Touch (All Levels)

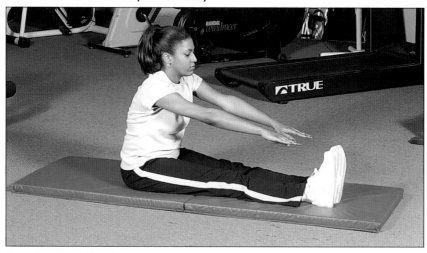

Bending from the hips, keep your back straight and reach for your toes; keep your knees slightly bent.

## ▼ Standing Lunge (Level 3)

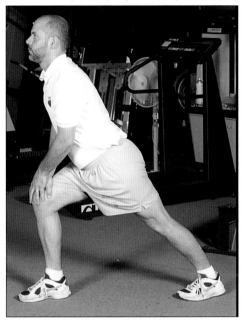

Point both feet forward and lean the front knee over but not past the front toe.

## ▼ Standing Hamstring Stretch (Level 3)

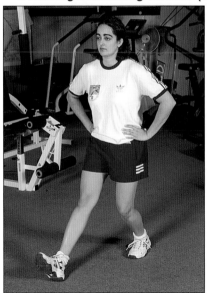 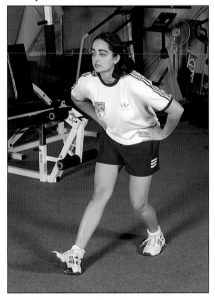

With one leg out straight and the other one bent slightly, slowly lean forward over the straight leg. Keep the back straight and the head up. Repeat with the other leg.

# ADDITIONAL EXERCISES

### ▼ Triceps Stretch (Arms and Shoulders)

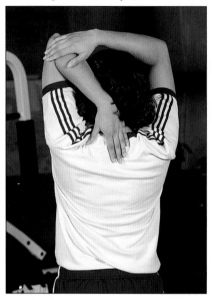 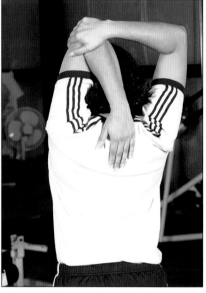

Place your left hand between your shoulder blades.

Use your right hand to gently push up and back at your left elbow, then switch sides.

### ▼ Lying Hamstring Stretch (Legs)

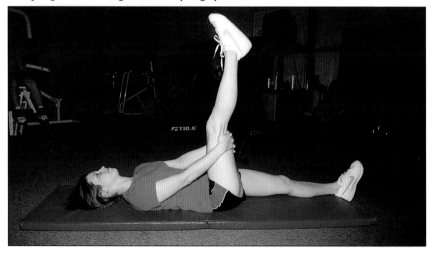

Lie flat, keeping both knees slightly bent as you gently pull one leg toward the chest and then the other.

## ▼ Elbow Cobra (Back)

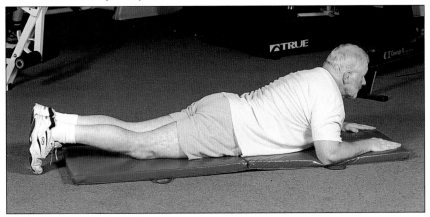

Keep your abdomen on the floor as you lift your upper body with your head and neck in a relaxed position.

## ▼ Butterfly (Legs)

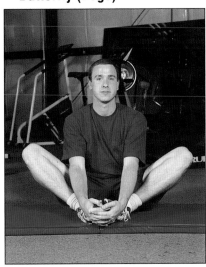 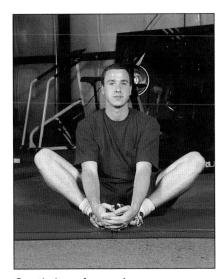

Hold the soles of your feet together.    Gently lean forward.

CHAPTER

# 6

# The ACSM Fitness Program

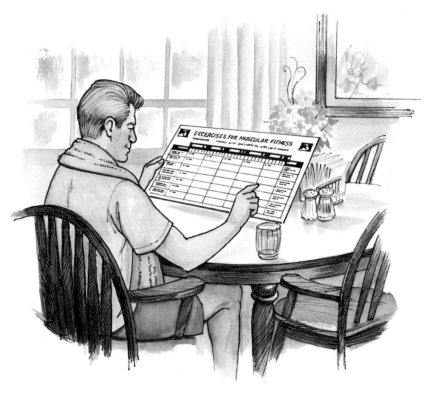

The ACSM Fitness Program is a personalized plan that allows you to exercise at the proper intensity for your own fitness level, which you discovered for each component of the ACSM Fitness Test—aerobic fitness, muscular fitness, flexibility, and body composition. In this chapter, we provide exercises that are appropriate for your level of fitness in each area.

# How It Works

First, review your personal fitness profile that we created from the results of the ACSM Fitness Test. Throughout this chapter, we will refer to the results of our models, Jackie and Frank. As with Jackie and Frank, you may be at different fitness levels in each of the four fitness areas. In the ACSM Fitness Program, you will select the exercise level that matches your fitness level for each fitness component. Our color coding makes this easy for you, because the exercise levels in the ACSM Fitness Program match the color coding from the ACSM Fitness Test, as indicated in this chart:

| Fitness Test Fitness Level | Color | Fitness Program Exercise Level |
|---|---|---|
| Low | Blue | 1 |
| Moderate | Green | 2 |
| Good | Yellow | 3 |
| High | Red | 4 |

Jackie recorded her ACSM Fitness Program results on page 87. Based on their test results, Frank's and Jackie's personal ACSM Fitness Program would include the following:

| | Frank | Jackie |
|---|---|---|
| Warm-up and aerobic fitness | Level 3 | Level 2 |
| Muscular fitness | Level 3 | Level 3 |
| Flexibility | Level 1 | Level 2 |
| Body composition | Level 3 | Level 4 |

# Putting Together Your Own Program

After reviewing your results from the ACSM Fitness Test, we can now plan your personal fitness program.

1. Refer to your ACSM Fitness Test results to check your fitness levels for each fitness component. Indicate each, and the color associated with it, in the following table.

| Fitness component | Fitness level | Color | Exercise level |
|---|---|---|---|
| Aerobic fitness | | | |
| Muscular fitness | | | |
| Flexibility | | | |
| Body composition | | | |

2. Based on the color code for your fitness level in each of the fitness components, determine the exercise level you should follow for each fitness component and mark it in the table. Here is how Jackie's chart looks:

| Fitness component | Fitness level | Color | Exercise level |
|---|---|---|---|
| Aerobic fitness | Below Average | Green | 2 |
| Muscular fitness | Average | Yellow | 3 |
| Flexibility | Below Average | Green | 2 |
| Body composition | Moderate Risk | Red | 4 |

3. Your personal ACSM Fitness Program includes the exercises indicated in each of the four components. Turn to the appropriate sections in the pages at the end of this chapter for lists of the specific exercises you will be doing. (You can refer back to chapter 5 if you need a reminder of how to do an exercise.)

4. We recommend that you perform the exercises in the order we present them. However, you can rearrange the sequence to fit your personal needs.

5. As you perform the exercises, record your progress in the exercise logs. Each time you exercise, write the date at the top of a new column. Check off the exercises you perform. It is a good idea to leave yourself notes about specific exercises. You can write in the margins or get a small notebook to record your comments. Frank's muscular fitness program looks like this:

| Date | Week 1 | | | | | | Week 2 | | | | | | Week 3 | | | | | |
|---|---|---|---|---|---|---|---|---|---|---|---|---|---|---|---|---|---|---|
| | 8/6 | 8/8 | | | | | | | | | | | | | | | | |
| **Single-Arm Row (p. 97)** | 8 each side | | | | | | 10 each side | | | | | | 12 each side | | | | | |
| | ✔ | ✔ | | | | | | | | | | | | | | | | |
| **Stair Step (p. 99)** | 8 each side | | | | | | 10 each side | | | | | | 12 each side | | | | | |
| | ✔ | ✔ | | | | | | | | | | | | | | | | |
| **Straight-Arm Curl-Up (p. 102)** | 8 times | | | | | | 10 times | | | | | | 12 times | | | | | |
| | ✔ | ✔ | | | | | | | | | | | | | | | | |
| **Knee Push-Up (p. 96)** | 6 times | | | | | | 18 times | | | | | | 11 times | | | | | |
| | ✔ | ✔ | | | | | | | | | | | | | | | | |
| **Prone Single-Leg Lift (p. 103)** | 6 each side | | | | | | 8 each side | | | | | | 11 each side | | | | | |
| | ✔ | ✔ | | | | | | | | | | | | | | | | |

6. Progress to a new time or number of repetitions when you have completed the time or number of repetitions indicated in that level. Continue to progress in the other exercises even if you must remain at a particular exercise for several days. You will develop your exercise program at your individual rate of progress. When you reach the end of week 6, continue with all exercises in the program until all of the exercises have caught up to the same level.

7. Once you have reached the end of your six-week program, it is time to reassess your fitness levels, repeating the ACSM Fitness Test procedures. A new exercise program can then be developed based on your new level of fitness. It will also show you how well you have progressed.

# Exercising Safely and Wisely

Most people, even those diagnosed with a chronic illness (with a physician's clearance) can exercise safely if some precautions are taken before, during, and after exercise. You can do the following both to ensure your safety while exercising and to maximize your health benefits. Regardless of your initial level of fitness, the following precautions should be observed:

• Drink extra fluids. Drink a glass full of water before you exercise and another after you have finished. Drink additional water every 15 to 20 minutes during exercise. Carry a bottle of water or sports beverage with you during your aerobic exercise if your exercise program exceeds 45 minutes. Many people like to drink a sports drink before and during exercise. Feel free to do this if you do not experience gastric distress.

• You do not need to take any extra vitamins or other supplements when exercising. A well-balanced diet provides most of the nutrients that a healthy, active person needs. Additional vitamins, proteins, amino acids, or other products are not usually necessary, and they typically do not improve your performance.

If you question the completeness of your diet, an inexpensive multi-vitamin/multi-mineral supplement may be a good idea.

• Follow your doctor's recommendations concerning any medications you may be taking. Special precautions should always be observed for anyone taking medication prescribed by a physician. While just about anyone can benefit from regular exercise, check with your doctor if you are taking medication and want to start an exercise program.

• Pay special attention to any discomfort you may feel during exercise. It is normal to feel a slight stiffness or soreness the day following your first or second exercise session. This discomfort should disappear in a day or two. However, if you experience any sudden pain while performing the exercises listed in your program, stop that exercise immediately and go on to the next one. During your next exercise session, try all the exercises again. If you still have pain or discomfort while doing a particular exercise, stop doing it until you consult with your doctor. Note that a pain or discomfort in the chest should not be ignored, because this could be an initial signal of developing heart disease. If upon exertion you feel a pain or tightness in the chest, consult your doctor right away for further evaluation before continuing your exercise program.

• Adjust your exercise regimen when you are not feeling well. When you are sick, your body needs its resources to fight off the illness. Take a few days off from your exercise program. If this time period is less than a week, you can resume your regular exercise program.

• On days when you are too busy to complete your exercise program, complete whatever portion you can, even if it is only 10 or 15 minutes. On days that you know are going to be busy, try to deliberately increase physical activity throughout the day. Remember that an accumulation of increased physical activity contributes to your overall health. An example might be to take the stairs instead of the elevator or to park your car farther from the front door.

# ACSM Fitness Programs and Logs

Now is the time to start using all the information you have gathered from your goals and your ACSM Fitness Test to begin your own ACSM Fitness Program. Everything you need to use the program is included on the program log sheets beginning on page 136. You will find the exercises you need to do, the time or suggested number of repetitions for each exercise, and a place to record your accomplishments. Do not forget to warm up before you begin the exercise program. Remember that body composition improves as you do aerobic and muscular fitness exercises. Increasing the frequency of your exercise program will help to increase lean body weight and reduce fat weight, contributing to a more favorable body composition.

# Recommendations

You should exercise based on your personal body composition assessments.

For example, if you are:

• **Level 1, Blue**—Your body composition assessments indicate that the amount of body fat you have may be too low. We recommend that you consult your doctor before beginning an exercise program.

• **Level 2, Green**—Your body composition assessments indicate that the amount of body fat you have may be too high. We recommend that you exercise four to six days per week for aerobic fitness, at least three days per week for flexibility, and two to three days per week for muscular fitness.

• **Level 3, Yellow**—Your body composition assessments indicate that the amount of body fat you have is moderate. We recommend that you do aerobic and flexibility exercises three to five days a week and muscular fitness exercises two to three days per week.

• **Level 4, Red**—Your body composition assessments indicate that the amount of body fat you have is good. We recommend that you do aerobic and flexibility exercises three to five days per week, and muscular fitness exercises two to three days per week.

# LEVEL 1

## Exercises for
## Warm-Up and Aerobic Fitness

**Equipment:** Stopwatch or watch with a second hand

| | Week 1 | Week 2 | Week 3 |
|---|---|---|---|
| **Date** | | | |
| **Shoulder Rolls (p. 110)** | 3 backward, 3 forward | 3 backward, 3 forward | 3 backward, 3 forward |
| **Head Tilt (p. 109)** | 10 sec 2 times | 10 sec 2 times | 10 sec 2 times |
| **Walk in Place** | 2 min | 2 min | 2 min |
| **Side Reach (p. 113)** | 5 each side | 5 each side | 5 each side |
| **Standing Cat Stretch (p. 112)** | 10 sec 2 times | 10 sec 2 times | 10 sec 2 times |
| **Chest Stretch (p. 112)** | 10 sec each side | 10 sec each side | 10 sec each side |
| **Wall Lean (p. 115)** | 10 sec each side | 10 sec each side | 10 sec each side |
| **Quadriceps Stretch (p. 116)** | 10 sec each side | 10 sec each side | 10 sec each side |
| **Walking** | 10 min: 5 out and back | 10 min: 6 out and back | 10 min: 7:30 out and back |

# LEVEL 1

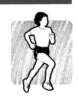

| Week 4 | Week 5 | Week 6 | Date |
|---|---|---|---|
| 3 backward, 3 forward | 3 backward, 3 forward | 3 backward, 3 forward | **Shoulder Rolls (p. 110)** |
| 10 sec 2 times | 10 sec 2 times | 10 sec 2 times | **Head Tilt (p. 109)** |
| 2 min | 2 min | 2 min | **Walk in Place** |
| 7 each side | 8 each side | 10 each side | **Side Reach (p. 113)** |
| 15 sec 2 times | 15 sec 2 times | 15 sec 2 times | **Standing Cat Stretch (p. 112)** |
| 15 sec each side | 15 sec each side | 15 sec each side | **Chest Stretch (p. 112)** |
| 15 sec each side | 15 sec each side | 15 sec each side | **Wall Lean (p. 115)** |
| 15 sec each side | 15 sec each side | 15 sec each side | **Quadriceps Stretch (p. 116)** |
| 15 min: 8 out, 7 back (Walk faster back.) | 20 min: 10 out, 10 back | 20 min: 10 out, 10 back (Walk farther each day.) | **Walking** |

# LEVEL 2

## Exercises for
## Warm-Up and Aerobic Fitness

**Equipment:** Stopwatch or watch with a second hand

| | Week 1 | Week 2 | Week 3 |
|---|---|---|---|
| **Date** | | | |
| **Shoulder Rolls (p. 110)** | 5 backward, 5 forward | 5 backward, 5 forward | 5 backward, 5 forward |
| **Head Turn (p. 109)** | 5 sec each side 2 times | 5 sec each side 2 times | 5 sec each side 2 times |
| **Walk in Place** | 2 min | 2 min | 2 min |
| **Side Reach (p. 113)** | 10 each side | 10 each side | 10 each side |
| **Standing Cat Stretch (p. 112)** | 15 sec 2 times | 15 sec 2 times | 15 sec 2 times |
| **Chest Stretch (p. 112)** | 15 sec each side | 15 sec each side | 15 sec each side |
| **Shoulder Stretch (p. 111)** | 15 sec each side | 15 sec each side | 15 sec each side |
| **Wall Lean (p. 115)** | 15 sec each side | 15 sec each side | 15 sec each side |
| **Seated Toe Touch (p. 116)** | 15 sec 2 times | 15 sec 2 times | 15 sec 2 times |
| **Walking** | 20 min: 10 out and 10 back | 20 min: 10 out, 10 back (Walk farther each day.) | 25 min: 12:30 out and back |

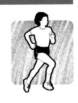

| Week 4 | Week 5 | Week 6 | Date |
|---|---|---|---|
| | | | **Date** |
| 5 backward, 5 forward | 5 backward, 5 forward | 5 backward, 5 forward | **Shoulder Rolls (p. 110)** |
| 10 sec each side 2 times | 10 sec each side 2 times | 10 sec each side 2 times | **Head Turn (p. 109)** |
| 2 min | 2 min | 2 min | **Walk in Place** |
| 12 each side | 13 each side | 15 each side | **Side Reach (p. 113)** |
| 15 sec 3 times | 15 sec 3 times | 15 sec 3 times | **Standing Cat Stretch (p. 112)** |
| 20 sec each side | 20 sec each side | 20 sec each side | **Chest Stretch (p. 112)** |
| 20 sec each side | 20 sec each side | 20 sec each side | **Shoulder Stretch (p. 111)** |
| 20 sec each side | 20 sec each side | 20 sec each side | **Wall Lean (p. 115)** |
| 20 sec 2 times | 20 sec 2 times | 20 sec 2 times | **Seated Toe Touch (p. 116)** |
| 25 min: 13 out, 12 back (Walk faster back.) | 30 min: 15 out and back | 30 min: 15 out and back (Walk farther each day.) | **Walking** |

# LEVEL 3

## Exercises for Warm-Up and Aerobic Fitness

**Equipment:** Stopwatch or watch with a second hand

| | Week 1 | Week 2 | Week 3 |
|---|---|---|---|
| **Date** | | | |
| **Head Tilt** (p. 109) | 10 sec 2 times | 10 sec 2 times | 10 sec 2 times |
| **Head Lean** (p. 110) | 10 sec each side | 10 sec each side | 10 sec each side |
| **Walk in Place** | 2 min | 2 min | 2 min |
| **Arm Circles** (p. 111) | 5 forward, 5 backward | 5 forward, 5 backward | 5 forward, 5 backward |
| **Standing Cat Stretch** (p. 112) | 15 sec 3 times | 15 sec 3 times | 15 sec 3 times |
| **Shoulder Turn** (p. 113) | 15 sec each side | 15 sec each side | 15 sec each side |
| **Chest Stretch** (p. 112) | 20 sec each side | 20 sec each side | 20 sec each side |
| **Standing Lunge** (p. 117) | 15 sec each side | 15 sec each side | 15 sec each side |
| **Standing Hamstring Stretch** (p. 117) | 15 sec each side | 15 sec each side | 15 sec each side |
| **Walking** | 30 min: 15 out and back | 30 min: 15 out and back (Walk farther each day.) | 35 min: 17:30 out and back |

| Week 4 | Week 5 | Week 6 | Date |
|---|---|---|---|
| | | | |
| 10 sec<br>2 times | 10 sec<br>2 times | 10 sec<br>2 times | **Head Tilt<br>(p. 109)** |
| 10 sec each side | 10 sec each side | 10 sec each side | **Head Lean<br>(p. 110)** |
| 2 min | 2 min | 2 min | **Walk in Place** |
| 7 forward,<br>7 backward | 8 forward,<br>8 backward | 10 forward,<br>10 backward | **Arm Circles<br>(p. 111)** |
| 15 sec<br>3 times | 15 sec<br>3 times | 15 sec<br>3 times | **Standing Cat<br>Stretch (p. 112)** |
| 20 sec<br>each side | 20 sec<br>each side | 20 sec<br>each side | **Shoulder Turn<br>(p. 113)** |
| 20 sec<br>each side | 20 sec<br>each side | 20 sec<br>each side | **Chest Stretch<br>(p. 112)** |
| 20 sec<br>each side | 20 sec<br>each side | 20 sec<br>each side | **Standing Lunge<br>(p. 117)** |
| 20 sec<br>each side | 20 sec<br>each side | 20 sec<br>each side | **Standing<br>Hamstring<br>Stretch (p. 117)** |
| 35 min:<br>18 out, 17 back<br>(Walk faster<br>back.) | 40 min:<br>20 out and back | 40 min:<br>20 out and back<br>(Walk farther<br>each day.) | **Walking** |

# LEVEL 4

## Exercises for
## Warm-Up and Aerobic Fitness

**Equipment:** Stopwatch or watch with a second hand

| | Week 1 | Week 2 | Week 3 |
|---|---|---|---|
| **Date** | | | |
| **Shoulder Rolls** (p. 110) | 5 backward, 5 forward | 5 backward, 5 forward | 5 backward, 5 forward |
| **Head Tilt** (p. 109) | 10 sec 2 times | 10 sec 2 times | 10 sec 2 times |
| **Head Turn** (p. 109) | 10 sec each side 2 times | 10 sec each side 2 times | 10 sec each side 2 times |
| **Walk in Place** | 2 min | 2 min | 2 min |
| **Side Reach** (p. 113) | 5 each side | 5 each side | 5 each side |
| **Standing Cat Stretch** (p. 112) | 10 sec 2 times | 10 sec 2 times | 10 sec 2 times |
| **Chest Stretch** (p. 112) | 10 sec each side | 10 sec each side | 10 sec each side |
| **Wall Lean** (p. 115) | 10 sec each side | 10 sec each side | 10 sec each side |
| **Quadriceps Stretch** (p. 116) | 10 sec each side | 10 sec each side | 10 sec each side |
| **Walking** | 40 min: 20 out and back | 40 min: 20 out and back (Walk farther each day.) | 40 min: 20:30 out, 19:30 back (Walk faster back.) |

| Week 4 | Week 5 | Week 6 | Date |
|--------|--------|--------|------|
| 5 backward, 5 forward | 5 backward, 5 forward | 5 backward, 5 forward | **Shoulder Rolls (p. 110)** |
| 10 sec 2 times | 10 sec 2 times | 10 sec 2 times | **Head Tilt (p. 109)** |
| 10 sec each side 2 times | 10 sec each side 2 times | 10 sec each side 2 times | **Head Turn (p. 109)** |
| 2 min | 2 min | 2 min | **Walk in Place** |
| 7 each side | 7 each side | 7 each side | **Side Reach (p. 113)** |
| 15 sec 2 times | 15 sec 2 times | 15 sec 2 times | **Standing Cat Stretch (p. 112)** |
| 15 sec each side | 15 sec each side | 15 sec each side | **Chest Stretch (p. 112)** |
| 15 sec each side | 15 sec each side | 15 sec each side | **Wall Lean (p. 115)** |
| 15 sec each side | 15 sec each side | 15 sec each side | **Quadriceps Stretch (p. 116)** |
| 45 min: 22:30 out and back | 45 min: 23 out, 22 back (Walk faster back.) | 45 min: Find a pleasant loop, rather than an out and back path. | **Walking** |

# LEVEL 1

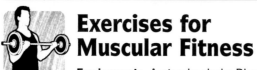

## Exercises for Muscular Fitness

**Equipment:** A sturdy chair; Plastic jugs partially filled with water or sand.

| Date | Week 1 | Week 2 | Week 3 |
|---|---|---|---|
| **Wall Push-Up (p. 94)** | 4 times | 6 times | 8 times |
| **Single-Arm Row (p. 97)** | 4 each side | 6 each side | 8 each side |
| **Seated Lower Leg Lift (p. 98)** | 4 each side | 6 each side | 8 each side |
| **Neck Curl-up (p. 101)** | 4 times | 6 times | 8 times |

| Week 4 | Week 5 | Week 6 | Date |
|--------|--------|--------|------|
| | | | |
| 11 times | 13 times | 15 times | **Wall Push-Up (p. 94)** |
| | | | |
| 11 each side | 13 each side | 15 each side | **Single-Arm Row (p. 97)** |
| | | | |
| 11 each side | 13 each side | 15 each side | **Seated Lower Leg Lift (p. 98)** |
| | | | |
| 11 times | 13 times | 15 times | **Neck Curl-Up (p. 101)** |
| | | | |

# LEVEL 2

## Exercises for Muscular Fitness

**Equipment:** A sturdy chair; Plastic jugs partially filled with water or sand.

| | Week 1 | Week 2 | Week 3 |
|---|---|---|---|
| **Date** | | | |
| **Chair Push-Up** (p. 95) | 4 times | 5 times | 6 times |
| **Toe Raise** (p. 100) | 4 times | 5 times | 6 times |
| **Seated Straight-Leg Lift (p. 99)** | 6 each side | 8 each side | 11 each side |
| **Single-Arm Row** (p. 97) | 6 each side | 8 each side | 11 each side |
| **Shoulder Curl-Up (p. 101)** | 6 times | 8 times | 11 times |
| **Prone Neck Lift (p. 103)** | 4 times | 5 times | 6 times |

# LEVEL 2

| Week 4 | Week 5 | Week 6 | Date |
|--------|--------|--------|------|
| 8 times | 11 times | 15 times | **Chair Push-Up (p. 95)** |
| 8 times | 11 times | 15 times | **Toe Raise (p. 100)** |
| 14 each side | 17 each side | 20 each side | **Seated Straight-Leg Lift (p. 99)** |
| 14 each side | 17 each side | 20 each side | **Single-Arm Row (p. 97)** |
| 14 times | 17 times | 20 times | **Shoulder Curl-Up (p. 101)** |
| 8 times | 11 times | 15 times | **Prone Neck Lift (p. 103)** |

# Exercises for Muscular Fitness

**Equipment:** A bench or step 8 to 12 inches high; Plastic jugs partially filled with water or sand.

| | Week 1 | | | | Week 2 | | | | Week 3 | | | |
|---|---|---|---|---|---|---|---|---|---|---|---|---|
| **Date** | | | | | | | | | | | | |
| **Single-Arm Row (p. 97)** | 8 each side | | | | 10 each side | | | | 12 each side | | | |
| **Stair Step (p. 99)** | 8 each side | | | | 10 each side | | | | 12 each side | | | |
| **Straight-Arm Curl-Up (p. 102)** | 8 times | | | | 10 times | | | | 12 times | | | |
| **Knee Push-Up (p. 96)** | 6 times | | | | 8 times | | | | 11 times | | | |
| **Prone Single-Leg Lift (p. 103)** | 6 each side | | | | 8 each side | | | | 11 each side | | | |

| Week 4 | Week 5 | Week 6 | Date |
|---|---|---|---|
| 14 each side | 17 each side | 20 each side | **Single-Arm Row (p. 97)** |
| 14 each side | 17 each side | 20 each side | **Stair Step (p. 99)** |
| 14 times | 17 times | 20 times | **Straight-Arm Curl-Up (p. 102)** |
| 14 times | 17 times | 20 times | **Knee Push-Up (p. 96)** |
| 14 each side | 17 each side | 20 each side | **Prone Single-Leg Lift (p. 103)** |

# LEVEL 4

 ## Exercises for Muscular Fitness

**Equipment:** A sturdy chair; Plastic jugs partially filled with water or sand.

| | Week 1 | Week 2 | Week 3 |
|---|---|---|---|
| **Date** | | | |
| **Biceps Curl** (p. 97) | 6 each side | 8 each side | 11 each side |
| **Reverse Fly** (p. 98) | 6 each side | 8 each side | 11 each side |
| **Chair Squat** (p. 100) | 6 times | 8 times | 11 times |
| **Toe Raise** (p. 100) | 6 each side | 8 each side | 11 each side |
| **Toe Push-Up** (p. 96) | 6 times | 8 times | 11 times |
| **Prone Head- and Leg-Lift** (p. 104) | 6 each side | 8 each side | 11 each side |
| **Crossed-Arm Curl-Up** (p. 102) | 8 times | 10 times | 12 times |

# LEVEL 4

| Week 4 | Week 5 | Week 6 | Date |
|--------|--------|--------|------|
| 14 each side | 17 each side | 20 each side | **Biceps Curl** (p. 97) |
| 14 each side | 17 each side | 20 each side | **Reverse Fly** (p. 98) |
| 14 times | 17 times | 20 times | **Chair Squat** (p. 100) |
| 14 each side | 17 each side | 20 each side | **Toe Raise** (p. 100) |
| 14 times | 17 times | 20 times | **Toe Push-Up** (p. 96) |
| 14 each side | 17 each side | 20 each side | **Prone Head- and Leg-Lift** (p. 104) |
| 14 times | 17 times | 20 times | **Crossed-Arm Curl-Up** (p. 102) |

# LEVEL 1

## Exercises for
## Flexibility and Cool-Down

**Equipment:** Watch or clock with a second hand

|  | Week 1 | Week 2 | Week 3 |
|---|---|---|---|
| **Date** | | | |
| **Shoulder Rolls (p. 110)** | 3 backward, 3 forward | 3 backward, 3 forward | 3 backward, 3 forward |
| **Chest Stretch (p. 112)** | 10 sec each side 2 times | 10 sec each side 2 times | 15 sec each side 2 times |
| **Wall Lean (p. 115)** | 10 sec each side 2 times | 10 sec each side 2 times | 15 sec each side 2 times |
| **Quadriceps Stretch (p. 116)** | 10 sec each side 2 times | 10 sec each side 2 times | 15 sec each side 2 times |
| **Seated Toe Touch (p. 116)** | 10 sec 2 times | 10 sec 2 times | 15 sec 2 times |
| **Long Lying Stretch (p. 114)** | 10 sec 2 times | 10 sec 2 times | 10 sec 2 times |

| Week 4 | Week 5 | Week 6 | Date |
|---|---|---|---|
| 3 backward, 3 forward | 3 backward, 3 forward | 3 backward, 3 forward | **Shoulder Rolls (p. 110)** |
| 15 sec each side 2 times | 20 sec each side 2 times | 20 sec each side 2 times | **Chest Stretch (p. 112)** |
| 15 sec each side 2 times | 20 sec each side 2 times | 20 sec each side 2 times | **Wall Lean (p. 115)** |
| 15 sec each side 2 times | 20 sec each side 2 times | 20 sec each side 2 times | **Quadriceps Stretch (p. 116)** |
| 15 sec 2 times | 20 sec 2 times | 20 sec 2 times | **Seated Toe Touch (p. 116)** |
| 10 sec 2 times | 10 sec 2 times | 10 sec 2 times | **Long Lying Stretch (p. 114)** |

# LEVEL 2

## Exercises for Flexibility and Cool-Down

**Equipment:** Watch or clock with a second hand

| | Week 1 | Week 2 | Week 3 |
|---|---|---|---|
| **Date** | | | |
| **Shoulder Rolls (p. 110)** | 5 backward, 5 forward | 5 backward, 5 forward | 5 backward, 5 forward |
| **Chest Stretch (p. 112)** | 20 sec each side 2 times | 20 sec each side 2 times | 20 sec each side 2 times |
| **Wall Lean (p. 115)** | 20 sec each side 2 times | 20 sec each side 2 times | 20 sec each side 2 times |
| **Quadriceps Stretch (p. 116)** | 20 sec each side 2 times | 20 sec each side 2 times | 20 sec each side 2 times |
| **Seated Toe Touch (p. 116)** | 20 sec 2 times | 20 sec 2 times | 20 sec 2 times |
| **Single-Knee to Chest Stretch (p. 114)** | 10 sec each side 2 times | 10 sec each side 2 times | 15 sec each side 2 times |
| **Long Lying Stretch (p. 114)** | 15 sec 2 times | 15 sec 2 times | 15 sec 2 times |

# LEVEL 2

| Week 4 | Week 5 | Week 6 | Date |
|--------|--------|--------|------|
| 5 backward, 5 forward | 5 backward, 5 forward | 5 backward, 5 forward | **Shoulder Rolls (p. 110)** |
| 20 sec each side 2 times | 20 sec each side 2 times | 20 sec each side 2 times | **Chest Stretch (p. 112)** |
| 20 sec each side 2 times | 20 sec each side 2 times | 20 sec each side 2 times | **Wall Lean (p. 115)** |
| 20 sec each side 2 times | 20 sec each side 2 times | 20 sec each side 2 times | **Quadriceps Stretch (p. 116)** |
| 20 sec 2 times | 20 sec 2 times | 20 sec 2 times | **Seated Toe Touch (p. 116)** |
| 15 sec each side 2 times | 20 sec each side 2 times | 20 sec each side 2 times | **Single-Knee to Chest Stretch (p. 114)** |
| 15 sec 2 times | 15 sec 2 times | 15 sec 2 times | **Long Lying Stretch (p. 114)** |

## Exercises for
## Flexibility and Cool-Down

**Equipment:** Watch or clock with a second hand

| | Week 1 | Week 2 | Week 3 |
|---|---|---|---|
| **Date** | | | |
| **Shoulder Rolls (p. 110)** | 5 backward, 5 forward | 5 backward, 5 forward | 5 backward, 5 forward |
| **Chest Stretch (p. 112)** | 20 sec each side 2 times | 20 sec each side 2 times | 20 sec each side 2 times |
| **Wall Lean (p. 115)** | 20 sec each side 2 times | 20 sec each side 2 times | 20 sec each side 2 times |
| **Quadriceps Stretch (p. 116)** | 20 sec each side 2 times | 20 sec each side 2 times | 20 sec each side 2 times |
| **Seated Toe Touch (p. 116)** | 20 sec 2 times | 20 sec 2 times | 20 sec 2 times |
| **Double-Knee to Chest Stretch (p. 115)** | 10 sec each side 2 times | 10 sec each side 2 times | 15 sec each side 2 times |
| **Long Lying Stretch (p. 114)** | 15 sec 2 times | 15 sec 2 times | 15 sec 2 times |

| Week 4 | Week 5 | Week 6 | Date |
|---|---|---|---|
| 5 backward, 5 forward | 5 backward, 5 forward | 5 backward, 5 forward | **Shoulder Rolls (p. 110)** |
| 20 sec each side 2 times | 20 sec each side 2 times | 20 sec each side 2 times | **Chest Stretch (p. 112)** |
| 20 sec each side 2 times | 20 sec each side 2 times | 20 sec each side 2 times | **Wall Lean (p. 115)** |
| 20 sec each side 2 times | 20 sec each side 2 times | 20 sec each side 2 times | **Quadriceps Stretch (p. 116)** |
| 20 sec 2 times | 20 sec 2 times | 20 sec 2 times | **Seated Toe Touch (p. 116)** |
| 15 sec each side 2 times | 20 sec each side 2 times | 20 sec each side 2 times | **Double-Knee to Chest Stretch (p. 115)** |
| 15 sec 2 times | 15 sec 2 times | 15 sec 2 times | **Long Lying Stretch (p. 114)** |

# LEVEL 4

## Exercises for Flexibility and Cool-Down

**Equipment:** Watch or clock with a second hand

| Date | Week 1 | Week 2 | Week 3 |
|---|---|---|---|
| Shoulder Rolls (p. 110) | 5 backward, 5 forward | 5 backward, 5 forward | 5 backward, 5 forward |
| Chest Stretch (p. 112) | 20 sec each side 2 times | 20 sec each side 2 times | 20 sec each side 2 times |
| Wall Lean (p. 115) | 20 sec each side 2 times | 20 sec each side 2 times | 20 sec each side 2 times |
| Quadriceps Stretch (p. 116) | 20 sec each side 2 times | 20 sec each side 2 times | 20 sec each side 2 times |
| Seated Toe Touch (p. 116) | 20 sec 2 times | 20 sec 2 times | 20 sec 2 times |
| Single-Knee to Chest Stretch (p. 114) | 10 sec each side 2 times | 10 sec each side 2 times | 15 sec each side 2 times |
| Double-Knee to Chest Stretch (p. 115) | 10 sec each side 2 times | 10 sec each side 2 times | 15 sec each side 2 times |
| Long Lying Stretch (p. 114) | 15 sec 2 times | 15 sec 2 times | 15 sec 2 times |

# LEVEL 4

| Week 4 | Week 5 | Week 6 | Date |
|---|---|---|---|
| 5 backward, 5 forward | 5 backward, 5 forward | 5 backward, 5 forward | **Shoulder Rolls (p. 110)** |
| 20 sec each side 2 times | 20 sec each side 2 times | 20 sec each side 2 times | **Chest Stretch (p. 112)** |
| 20 sec each side 2 times | 20 sec each side 2 times | 20 sec each side 2 times | **Wall Lean (p. 115)** |
| 20 sec each side 2 times | 20 sec each side 2 times | 20 sec each side 2 times | **Quadriceps Stretch (p. 116)** |
| 20 sec 2 times | 20 sec 2 times | 20 sec 2 times | **Seated Toe Touch (p. 116)** |
| 15 sec each side 2 times | 20 sec each side 2 times | 20 sec each side 2 times | **Single-Knee to Chest Stretch (p. 114)** |
| 15 sec each side 2 times | 20 sec each side 2 times | 20 sec each side 2 times | **Double-Knee to Chest Stretch (p. 115)** |
| 15 sec 2 times | 15 sec 2 times | 15 sec 2 times | **Long Lying Stretch (p. 114)** |

CHAPTER

# 7

# Staying Active

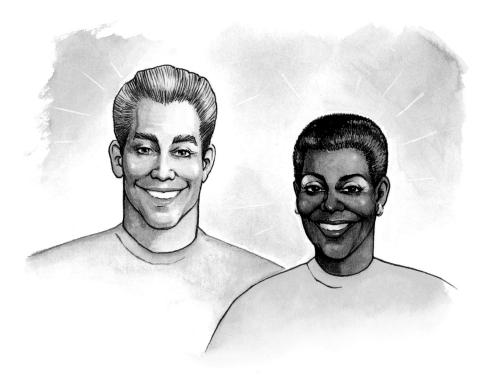

By the time you read this chapter, you will have completed about six weeks, or one level, of the ACSM Fitness Program. It is time to reassess your current fitness status and reevaluate your goals. Return to the assessments in the ACSM Fitness Test and reevaluate yourself. Then, review the fitness goals you identified earlier. Your fitness test results will show how you have progressed toward your goals.

Our model, Jackie, has met her first goal of being able to walk three miles without stopping, but she is not quite at her body mass index (BMI) goal. Our other model, Frank, is now able to reach 7 inches (17.8 centimeters) in the sit-and-reach test, which shows that his flexibility is improving. Both our models have made significant progress in their fitness and are achieving a healthier lifestyle.

Are you making progress toward your goals? Have you established new goals for your personal fitness program? If your goals continue to indicate that you would like to improve your fitness in one or more areas, then use the results of your updated assessment as a guide for selecting a new exercise level in each of the fitness components of the ACSM Fitness Program. Many of the exercises will be familiar to you, but you will also notice some new exercises at the next level. Or, do you need some motivation to change your current behavior to make it more conducive to a healthier lifestyle? This chapter provides you with information on how to continue your active lifestyle, motivational techniques to keep you going, and ways to make permanent changes in your behavior. It also includes ways to choose a commercial fitness facility and to purchase exercise equipment.

# Maintaining Motivation

Health club managers and exercise rehabilitation program staff have observed that about half of the people who join programs drop out within the first year. Even motivated patients with diagnosed heart disease exhibit this same drop-out rate. Recently published guidelines from the American College of Sports Medicine suggest several motivational strategies to improve adherence to healthy lifestyle programs.

# Start With a Moderate Exercise Program

Little additional benefits are to be gained with a high-intensity exercise program. In fact, the higher the intensity, the greater the chance of developing an orthopedic or cardiac complication. People who have just started an exercise program will experience some muscular discomfort the following day. However, beginning the program at a lower intensity reduces this muscular soreness. Eventually, the soreness will go away and will not return if the intensity is kept to a moderate level. The same holds true for increasing the frequency and the duration of the exercise program. We suggest that you first increase the number of days per week you exercise, then increase the duration before increasing the intensity. For most people, exercising at a lower intensity for a longer period of time is better than exercising at a higher intensity for a shorter period of time. Exercising at a lower intensity may improve your fitness, and it offers several advantages over exercise at a higher intensity:

- Decreases your risk of orthopedic problems
- Lowers the risk of cardiovascular complications
- Increases the likelihood of continuing the fitness program over a long time

Maintaining increased physical activity through your daily tasks is also essential for continued weight loss, if weight loss is included in your set of goals. In addition to your regular exercise program, you can increase daily activity in many ways, including the following:

- Walking rather than driving to complete short errands
- Deliberately parking farther from an entrance than you need to
- Leaving home a few minutes early to allow yourself time for a short walk before starting the work day
- Taking a short walk during coffee breaks or at lunch time
- Using stairs rather than elevators or escalators for climbs of several stories
- Doing your own lawn work, gardening, or housework
- Carrying a few packages to your car rather than using the shopping cart
- Walking your pet
- Scheduling play time with your children or grandchildren
- Walking rather than using a cart on the golf course

# Exercise With Others

Scientific evidence amply shows that participation in a structured exercise program will help maintain and improve your health. Motivation comes from being a part of the group. There is a poorer compliance rate when the exercise program is carried out alone. Join a health club, or recruit your family and friends to exercise with you. That way you can support each other.

Exercising with a group can be fun, and therefore more motivating and beneficial. Sometimes, exercising with other people is such fun that you are more likely to continue your fitness program with others than alone. At other times, exercising by yourself allows you to complete your exercise program at your own pace without being viewed or judged by others. Most aerobic activities can be done alone or with a group, whereas others, for safety reasons, are best done with a group.

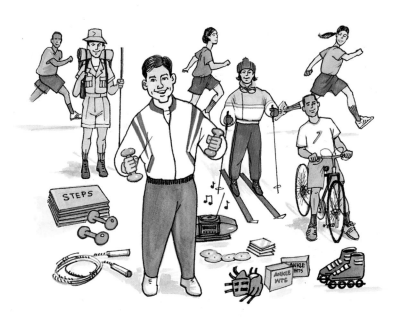

# Try Variety in Your Exercise Program

Many activities will improve your aerobic and muscular fitness. For aerobic fitness, activities other than walking that use large muscle groups in a continuous, rhythmic fashion will provide similar results. In addition to walking, jogging, or running, the following are some good aerobic activities and approximately how many calories they require during 30 minutes of exercise.

| Activity | Calories used in 30 minutes | |
|---|---|---|
| | 140 lb person (63.6 kg) | 180 lb person (81.8 kg) |
| Bicycling—10 mph (16 kph) | 200 | 260 |
| Cross-country skiing | 260 | 350 |
| Dancing—aerobic, moderate | 200 | 260 |
| Dancing—ballroom, leisure | 130 | 170 |
| Hiking | 160 | 200 |
| Ice skating, moderate | 230 | 300 |
| In-line skating | 230 | 300 |
| Jogging, 12 min per mile (7.5 min per km) | 260 | 350 |
| Rope skipping, 80 per min | 330 | 430 |
| Rowing, moderate | 230 | 300 |
| Running—6 min per mile (3.7 min per km) | 545 | 700 |
| Stair climbing | 260 | 350 |
| Swimming—freestyle, moderate | 260 | 350 |
| Walking—15 min per mile (9.3 min per km) | 135 | 175 |

You can do any of these activities, or a mixture of them, through-out the week. To improve your aerobic fitness you simply need to do some form of aerobic activity at least three days a week, but preferably most days of the week. Remember that to main-tain good health, it is most important to stay active, in whatever forms that activity may take. Because increasing the amount of physical activity in your daily life is so important to your health, you should choose one or several activities that you really en-joy and will look forward to in the future. Even if the activities you choose do not seem to provide as difficult a workout as other activities, you are more likely to continue exercising when you enjoy what you are doing. Selecting more than one activity and rotating the activities regularly will help prevent boredom and increase the likelihood of maintaining your exercise program. When selecting other kinds of exercise, you should consider several factors when choosing an aerobic activity for your per-sonal fitness program.

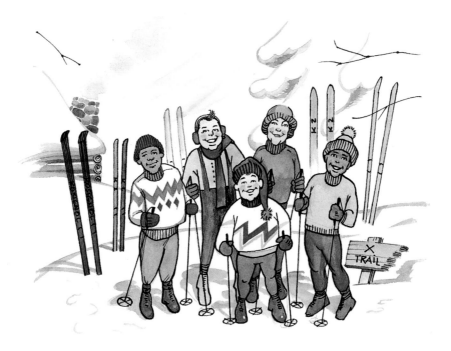

## Impact

Some aerobic activities, such as skipping rope, running, and some forms of aerobics, involve jumping and pounding that may be uncomfortable or lead to an acute injury or develop into a chronic one. Swimming, cross-country skiing, in-line skating, cycling, and rowing are easier on the joints. Select an exercise that you not only enjoy, but you also find comfortable. As you begin to become accustomed to regular exercise, then begin to explore other options that may require a higher level of fitness or increased muscular involvement.

## Convenience

Some aerobic activities require expensive equipment, are seasonal, or are not available in certain geographic locations. For example, it is difficult to make cross-country skiing a regular part of your fitness routine if it seldom snows where you live.

## Skill

Activities that require a lot of skill may be discouraging. It takes a while to learn to use in-line skates, for example. Many people stop exercising before they have developed the skills they need for the activity to become enjoyable.

# Establish a Routine and Chart Your Progress

We introduced you to Exercise Logs in chapter 6. Incorporated within these logs was an opportunity to write down your progress. You could then see how well you progressed throughout the initial stages of your new exercise program. You can continue to record your progress even after the initial stages of your program. Progress charts can also be a powerful motivator. For example, you can record your mileage if you walk, jog, or cycle. You can set as a goal either a certain number of miles or a certain distance. Then, you can reward yourself when you achieve the desired distance. Some people have used maps as well as progress charts. Each time a distance is completed, it is marked on the map. Your goal could include the distance between cities, between relatives' homes, or between parts of the country.

# Making Permanent Changes

Exercise professionals recognize that you must take into consideration two very important facts when making permanent changes in your lifestyle. First, exercise is voluntary. No one is forcing you to include exercise in your life. Second, exercise is time consuming. In our already busy lives, these two factors can easily be enough to interfere with your regular program. The suggestions we have made will, hopefully, provide you with incentives to include exercise and proper nutrition in your lifestyle so that they do not become a burden on your time.

In chapter 3, you learned how to set goals and manage your time to include a regular program of physical activity. Periodically, check your goals against your Exercise Logs and Program Charts to match your progress against your goals. If you have not reached your goals in the specified period of time or number of exercise sessions, evaluate your goals and reestablish your commitment. Here are some additional tips from exercise program experts:

- Set short- and long-term, realistic, and measurable goals.
- Remain confident you can achieve your goals.
- Write down a clear description of the goal and the means by which to achieve it.
- Get some feedback from a health and fitness expert, especially one certified by the ACSM.
- Revise your goals when appropriate.
- Develop a social support system that will provide you with encouragement and help during the difficult times.

## Guidelines for Healthy Aerobic Activity

- Exercise most days of the week (or about three to five times per week).
- Warm up for 5 to 10 minutes before aerobic activity.
- Maintain your exercise intensity for 20 to 60 minutes of continuous or intermittent (minimum of 10-minute bouts) activity accumulated throughout the day.
- Gradually decrease intensity and duration, then stretch to cool down during the last 5 to 10 minutes.
- If weight loss is a major goal, participate in your aerobic activity at least 30 minutes, five days per week.
- On days when you cannot complete your exercise program, complete whatever portion of it you can, even if it is only 10 or 15 minutes. In addition, deliberately increase physical activity throughout the day. Remember that all appropriate physical activity contributes to your overall health. Do not try to make up exercise sessions by cramming them all in on the weekend, by increasing the number of minutes of exercise in a single session, or by increasing the intensity of a session. This practice will only lead to injury.

# Choosing the Intensity of Aerobic Exercise

One very good way to determine whether you are exercising hard enough during your aerobic exercise is to measure your heart rate. First, calculate your exercise heart rate range using the steps in the following heart rate determination chart on page 162. Then, during your exercise, find your pulse at one of the places described in chapter 4. If your heart rate is within the range you have calculated, your intensity is at the appropriate level. For example, Frank's estimated maximum heart rate is 183 beats per minute (220 – 37, his age). By multiplying 183 by 0.6 and then by 0.9, Frank determined that his exercise heart rate range is between 110 and 165 beats per minute. Jackie's exercise heart rate range is between 103 and 155 beats per minute. The levels of 0.6 (60 percent) and 0.9 (90 percent) are rather arbitrary. Much of the scientific literature on exercise intensity shows that beginning exercisers do as well at lower intensities. Select a comfortable intensity. You can always increase the intensity later. Medications for high blood pressure or other conditions may affect your heart rate during exercise. Therefore, if you are taking such medications, consult your physician before determining your exercise heart rate range.

# Calculating Your Exercise Heart Rate Range

The following equations will help you calculate the intensity at which you should be exercising based on your heart rate.

1. Estimate your maximum heart rate.

    220 – age = _____ (maximum heart rate)

2. Determine your lower-limit exercise heart rate by multiplying your maximum heart rate by 0.6.

    Maximum heart rate _____ × 0.6 =

3. Determine your upper-limit exercise heart rate by multiplying your maximum heart rate by 0.9.

    Maximum heart rate _____ × 0.9 = _____

4. Your exercise heart rate range is between your lower (60 percent) and upper (90 percent) limits.

# Improving Muscular Fitness

Improving and progressing with your muscular fitness program can be as simple as continuing to do the exercises in the ACSM Fitness Program, but with heavier weights or more repetitions. In addition, you may want to join a fitness center or purchase home weight-training equipment. Regardless of the method you choose, follow these guidelines to ensure safe, effective exercise:

- Include exercises for each of the muscle areas shown in chapter 5.
- Complete 8 to 15 repetitions of each exercise. When you can easily complete 15 repetitions, increase the workload in either, or both, of these ways:
  a. Increase the amount of weight you lift.
  b. Do a second set of 8 to 15 repetitions.

# Commercial Fitness Facilities and Equipment

If you are ready for some additional variety in your exercise program, many opportunities are open to you, but caution is always advised before making a financial commitment when joining a commercial fitness club or purchasing new equipment. Many communities have various fitness centers or health clubs, and many stores offer exercise equipment, videos, and books. Consider the following guidelines for the selection and purchase of exercise equipment and when selecting a membership at a health club.

## Selecting Exercise Equipment

You may choose to expand your home exercise program by purchasing aerobic fitness or weight-training equipment. Exercising at home saves both the time and the expense of fitness center membership. It also allows you to exercise in privacy. However, health or fitness club membership can also be motivating.

Choosing the best equipment and programs may seem complicated and often appears to be expensive. Many different types of exercise equipment and programs are available for use in your home or at commercial fitness centers. Choices range from $20 collapsible equipment or videos to $10,000 state-of-the-art models. To add to the confusion, not all advertised products actually produce the desired results.

## Products to Avoid

Avoid a product if it makes any of the following claims. No exercise program or piece of equipment has been found to safely produce these results.

• "You will see results immediately!" Real improvements in your physical fitness or weight loss program take time. You may see minor changes in just a few days or weeks, but other, major changes may take longer. By regularly assessing your fitness using the ACSM Fitness Test, you will have a good indication of your personal progress.

• "This is an effortless, no-sweat workout!" If getting fit took no effort, everyone would be doing it. It takes effort and self-determination to improve your fitness. The ACSM Fitness Program is designed to help make your efforts more productive.

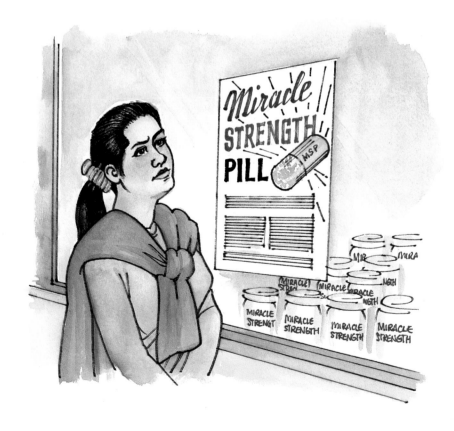

- "Lose fat from your thighs (or waist, or wherever); rid your-self of that cellulite!" No exercise can reduce fat specifically in the area exercised. During exercise, the body takes its energy from the fat stored all over your body. Cellulite is simply a name given to the dimpled fat that tends to accumulate on the hips and thighs of women and on the abdomen of men. Appropriate aerobic exercise will help reduce overall body fat and hence the cellulite appearance.

- "Wear this (vest, belt, or other special clothing) and lose inches off your waist and thighs!" Wearing "weight-reducing" cloth-ing or items such as these results in a temporary displacement of tissue or loss of water from the tissue, not a permanent loss of body fat. When you remove the item, the tissue soon regains its original shape; as soon as you drink, the water is replaced.

# Choosing Exercise Equipment and Programs Wisely

After reading this book and doing a little background work, com-mon sense on your part should allow you to select safe, effec-tive equipment that meets both your fitness needs and your budget. Whenever possible, try out any new equipment and pre-view any videos before you make a purchase. If you remain con-fused, consult an expert. Competent health and fitness experts are almost always certified by the ACSM.

Use the following checklists to help you decide which fitness equipment, health or fitness center, book, or video is right for you. Compare several items or clubs. Do not buy equipment just be-cause you have seen it advertised on television or because the salesperson says it is the best. Try it out to determine whether it feels right to you, whether you will use it, and whether you have room for it.

## *Selecting Equipment for Aerobic Fitness*

### *Comfort and Effectiveness*

- ✔ Is it easy to get onto and off of?
- ✔ Can it be adjusted to fit my body? (Check seat height, frame length, distance to foot rests, stride length, and handlebars, for instance.)

✔ Are there controls that allow me to adjust the workload?

✔ Is it comfortable enough that I could use it for 30 minutes or more?

### Reliability

✔ Can it support my weight?

✔ Is it sturdy, with a rigid frame that does not wobble when I use it?

✔ Are the gauges and controls easy to operate? What if they break?

### Ease of Use and Maintenance

✔ Can I assemble it, or will the dealer do it for me?

✔ Can I change the resistance or any of the settings easily? Will they stay where I put them?

✔ Where can I get the equipment repaired if it breaks?

### Cost

✔ How much does it cost?

✔ Does the price include shipping?

✔ Is there a warranty?

✔ Can I afford it?

✔ What are the alternatives if I do not buy it?

## Selecting Equipment for Muscular Fitness

### Comfort and Effectiveness

✔ Does the equipment fit my body?

✔ Can I adjust the weights so I can work with them as I progress from beginning to more advanced exercises?

✔ Are the exercise positions comfortable?

✔ Is the equipment padded where I want it to be?

✔ Does the equipment work all my muscles?

### Reliability

✔ Is the equipment sturdy (no wobbling or loose weights)?

✔ Do the weights move smoothly (no sticking or jerking)?

✔ Are additional weights or attachments available?

### Ease of Use and Maintenance

✔ Is it easy to assemble?

✔ Do I have to buy any special attachments or make adjustments to my home?

✔ Is it easy to change the weights?

✔ If it breaks, where can I get the equipment serviced or maintained?

### Cost

✔ What does it cost?

✔ Does the price include shipping?

✔ Is there a warranty?

✔ Can I afford it?

✔ What are the alternatives if I do not buy the equipment?

## Selecting a Health Club or Fitness Center

### Comfort and Convenience

✔ Is it close to my home or place of work?

✔ Are the hours convenient?

✔ Is day care available if I need it?

✔ Would I be comfortable exercising with the other clients?

✔ Will I make time to get to the center?

### Effectiveness

✔ Does it have all the equipment and services I want (treadmills, weights, pool, aerobics classes)?

✔ Is there enough equipment?

✔ Are locker facilities adequate?

✔ Is the staff friendly, knowledgeable, and available to assist me?

✔ Are the personnel certified? By what organization?

✔ Are new members given an orientation, including a fitness screening?

### Maintenance
- ✔ Is the facility clean, secure, and well ventilated?
- ✔ Is the equipment maintained?
- ✔ Are the safety and emergency procedures adequate?

### Cost
- ✔ Is there a trial or an introductory period?
- ✔ Can I afford the membership?
- ✔ Can I get my money back if I discontinue my membership?
- ✔ What are the alternatives if I do not join?

# Summary

Good nutrition and increased physical activity can and will increase both the quality and the quantity of your life. Increasing the amount of daily physical activity in your life is an important first step in your commitment to lead a healthy lifestyle. Good nutrition helps to reduce identified risk factors for many diseases. Earlier, we mentioned that incorporating a regular program of exercise was voluntary and time consuming. Now, we hope that you have come to realize that the time commitment is not that great and if you want to increase the quality (and the quantity) of your life, adding a program of regular physical activity is not really voluntary. We congratulate you on joining the ACSM Fitness Program and wish you good health as you continue with your lifelong commitment.

# Index

## K

kilocalorie. *see* calories
knee push-up, 96

## L

leg/hip exercises, 98–100
    butterfly stretch, 119
    inner-leg lift, 106
    outer leg lift, 107
    stretching, 116–119
level four exercises
    flexibility, 150–151
    muscular fitness, 142–143
    warm-up and aerobic fitness, 134–135
level one exercises
    flexibility, 144–145
    muscular fitness, 136–137
    warm-up and aerobic fitness, 128–129
level three exercises
    flexibility, 148–149
    muscular fitness, 140–141
    warm-up and aerobic fitness, 132–133
level two exercises
    flexibility, 146–147
    muscular fitness, 138–139
    warm-up and aerobic fitness, 130–131
life expectancy, 6–8
lifestyle changes, 160
limits and limitations, 51–52
long term goals, 44, 49–51
longevity, 6–8
low-density lipoprotein (LDL), 4
lungs, 5–6

## M

maximal oxygen consumption, 5
medical examination, 59
medications, 61, 126, 162
mental fitness, 43
metabolism, 22
missing a workout, 126
motivation
    and ambivalence, 55–56
    for beginning exercise program, 48
    defining, 52–53
    and guilt, 53–54
    internal vs. external, 53
    keys to mobilizing, 54
    and long term goals, 49–50
    maintaining, 14–17, 154
    and readiness for behavior change, 45
muscles
    and aerobic capacity, 6
    carbohydrates as fuel, 24
    fuel for activity, 20
    soreness and intensity of exercise, 15
    water/protein composition, 25
muscular fitness
    definition, 10
    general guidelines, 92–93
    guidelines, 162–163
    push-up test, 73–74
    selecting equipment, 166–167
    training principles, 93
muscular fitness exercises
    abdominal exercises, 101–102
    arms and shoulders, 94–98
    back exercises, 103–104
    biceps curl, 97
    chair push-up, 95
    inner-leg lift, 106

    knee push-up, 96
    lateral raise, 106
    leg/hip exercises, 98–100
    level four, 142–143
    level one, 136–137
    level three, 140–141
    level two exercises, 138–139
    outer leg lift, 107
    repetitions, 163
    reverse fly, 98
    shoulder shrugs, 106
    single-arm row, 97
    toe push up, 96
    wall push-up, 94

## N

neck stretches, 109–110
niacin, 30
"No pain, no gain.", 90
non-insulin-dependent diabetes. *see* diabetes
norms
    for push-up test, 74
    for sit and reach test, 77
    waist-to-hip ratio, 83
    for walking test, 68–71
nutrition
    and body composition, 27–29
    calcium, 31
    ergogenic aids, 33
    during exercise, 37–38
    hydration, 34–35
    interdependence with physical activity, 20
    iron, 31–32
    low carbohydrate diets, 24
    obesity in U.S. population, 20
    post-exercise, 38
    pre-exercise, 36–37
    protein requirements, 25–26
    timing of meals, 20–21
    vegetarian diet, 26
    vitamins, 29–31
    and weight control, 27–29
nutritional supplements
    ergogenic aids, 33
    and weight control, 28

## O

obesity, 20, 28
osteoporosis, 3, 4, 30
oxygen, 5, 32–33. *see also* aerobic capacity

## P

pain
    during exercise, 93, 126
    and fitness assessment participation, 61
    and flexibility, 108
    and intensity of exercise, 90
pantothenic acid, 30
persistence, 14
personal fitness profile
    evaluating score from walking test, 66–67
    matching exercise level and fitness level, 122–125
    sample results, 87
    steps to creating, 63–65
physical activity
    and caloric needs, 23
    CDC, Surgeon General, ACSM recommendations, 9
    and daily caloric requirements, 22–23
physical fitness. *see* fitness

# About the Writers

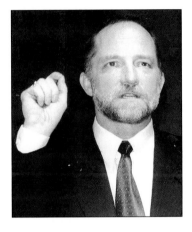

D r. Walter R. Thompson, PhD, FACSM, FAACVPR is a professor of kinesiology and health in the College of Education and a professor of nutrition in the College of Health and Human Sciences at Georgia State University in Atlanta. He is an ACSM Certified Program Director$_{SM}$, ACSM Registered Clinical Exercise Physiologist®, licensed Clinical Exercise Physiologist in the state of Louisiana, and licensed Clinical Laboratory Director in the state of Georgia. Before joining the faculty at Georgia State University, Dr. Thompson was a professor of health, human performance, and recreation at the University of Southern Mississippi and program director for the Center for Cardiac Rehabilitation and Health Enhancement at Swedish Covenant Hospital in Chicago. He has also held academic appointments at Northeastern Illinois University and George Williams College.

Dr. Thompson has been the chairman of the ACSM Committee on Certification and Education and is now the chairman of the ACSM International Relations Committee. He has given lectures on health-related topics in 20 different countries. He is a fellow of the American College of Sports Medicine, a fellow of the American Association for Cardiovascular and Pulmonary Rehabilitation, and a fellow of the Research Consortium of the American Alliance for Health, Physical Education, Recreation and Dance. He is also a member of the American Physiological Society and the American Public Health Association.

Dr. Thompson, his wife Deon, and their children Jessica and Aaron live in the suburbs of Atlanta, Georgia.

Dr. Dan Benardot, PhD, RD, FACSM, is associate professor of nutrition and associate professor of kinesiology and health at Georgia State University, and is co-director of the Laboratory for Elite Athlete Performance at GSU, which provides training and nutrition plans for competitive athletes seeking to enhance athletic performance. From 1984–1992 he served as chair of the department of nutrition, and from 1998–2002 he served as associate 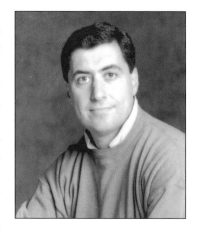 dean for research for the College of Health and Human Sciences at Georgia State University. He is a fellow of the American College of Sports Medicine, a registered and licensed dietitian, an officer of The United States Figure Skating Sports Medicine Society, and a member of the American Dietetic Association.

As the national team nutritionist and chair of the Athlete Wellness Program for USA Gymnastics, Benardot worked with the gold medal women's gymnastics team at the Atlanta Olympic Games in 1996, and was the first American to serve on the medical commission of Fédération International de Gymnastique (the international governing body for gymnastics.) Among numerous other published journal articles and book chapters, Benardot served as editor-in-chief for "Sports Nutrition: A Guide for the Professional Working with Active People" (2nd Edition), which was published by The American Dietetic Association, and authored *Nutrition for Serious Athletes*, which was published by Human Kinetics. He has received research funding from the United States Olympic Committee, The Gatorade Sports Science Institute, and The American Cancer Society.

Born in Salonika, Greece, Benardot gained his love for sport while growing up in the Lake Placid region of northern New York State. He now lives in Atlanta, Georgia with his wife and two children.

Dr. Steven Jonas, MD, MPH, MS, is professor of preventive medicine in the School of Medicine at State University of New York at Stony Brook. He is board certified in preventive medicine and is a fellow of the American College of Preventive Medicine.

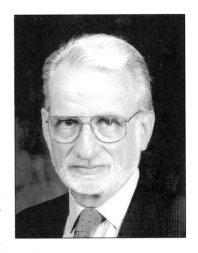

He has authored, coauthored, and edited more than 20 books, 12 of them on health, fitness, weight management, and wellness. The first of these was *Triathloning for Ordinary Mortals* (WW Norton, 1986, 1999). The most recent was *Talking About Health and Wellness With Patients: Integrating Health Promotion/Disease Prevention Into Your Practice* (Springer Publishing, 2000). He is a member of the editorial board of ACSM's Health & Fitness Journal.

In 2002, he began his 20th season of triathlon competition and is chairman of the Education Committee of the National Coaching Commission of USA Triathlon (the sport's national governing body). He is also a ski instructor, certified at Level I by the Professional Ski Instructors of America, and teaches skiing part-time at the Breckenridge Ski Resort in Colorado. Jonas currently resides in Stony Brook, New York.

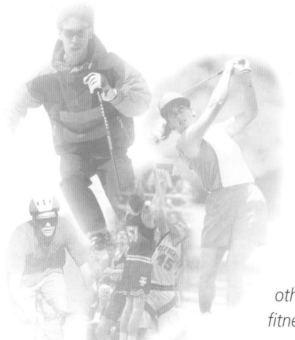

You'll find
other outstanding
fitness resources at

# www.HumanKinetics.com

In the U.S. call

## 800-747-4457

| | |
|---|---|
| Australia | 08 8277 1555 |
| Canada | 1-800-465-7301 |
| Europe | +44 (0) 113 255 5665 |
| New Zealand | 09-523-3462 |

**HUMAN KINETICS**
*The Premier Publisher for Sports and Fitness*
P.O. Box 5076 • Champaign, IL  61825-5076 USA